I0120468

Living Well with POTS, MCAS, and EDS

Evidence-Based Solutions for Managing
Postural Orthostatic Tachycardia Syndrome,
Mast Cell Activation Syndrome, and Ehlers-
Danlos Syndrome

Stella Marion Kaufman

Copyright © 2025 Stella Marion Kaufman. All rights reserved.

The information provided in "Living Well with POTS, MCAS, and EDS: Evidence-Based Solutions for Managing Postural Orthostatic Tachycardia Syndrome, Mast Cell Activation Syndrome, and Ehlers-Danlos Syndrome" is for educational and informational purposes only and is not intended as medical advice, diagnosis, or treatment.

This book does not:

- Replace professional medical consultation, examination, diagnosis, or treatment

- Provide specific medical recommendations for individual cases

- Constitute a doctor-patient relationship between the author and readers

- Guarantee specific health outcomes or treatment results

Readers should:

- Consult qualified healthcare professionals before making any medical decisions

- Discuss all symptoms, treatments, and management strategies with their medical team

- Seek immediate medical attention for emergency situations

- Continue all prescribed medications and treatments unless directed otherwise by their physicians

Postural Orthostatic Tachycardia Syndrome (POTS), Mast Cell Activation Syndrome (MCAS), and Ehlers-Danlos

Syndrome (EDS) are complex medical conditions that require individualized professional medical management. The strategies and information presented in this book represent general approaches and should be adapted to individual circumstances under professional medical supervision.

The author and publisher:

- Disclaim any liability for adverse effects or consequences resulting from the use of information contained herein

- Do not warrant the accuracy, completeness, or usefulness of any information provided

- Are not responsible for any errors or omissions in the content

Case Studies and Examples: The names and scenarios depicted in this book are fictitious and purely for illustrative purposes only. Any resemblance to actual persons, organisations, living or dead, or actual events is purely coincidental. Composite case studies have been created to protect patient privacy while demonstrating management principles.

Always consult with qualified healthcare professionals familiar with your specific medical history and current condition before implementing any suggestions from this book.

If you are experiencing a medical emergency, call emergency services immediately.

ISBN: 978-1-7641437-5-2
Isohan Publishing

Table of Contents

Preface

Living well with POTS, MCAS, and EDS—what many patients call "the trifecta"—can feel like navigating a medical maze without a map. When I began writing this guide, I encountered countless patients who described feeling lost in a healthcare system that often treats each condition separately, missing the profound connections between these three disorders. This book emerged from their stories, their struggles, and ultimately, their successes in creating meaningful lives alongside chronic illness.

Format and Approach

Each chapter begins with a narrative scenario featuring a composite patient facing real challenges that illustrate the chapter's key concepts. These opening stories serve multiple purposes: they demonstrate how theoretical concepts apply in daily life, provide emotional connection to the material, and offer hope through examples of successful problem-solving.

The content progresses logically from understanding your conditions through building your medical team, developing practical management strategies, and ultimately creating a fulfilling life that accommodates chronic illness realities. Each section includes specific, actionable guidance rather than general suggestions, recognizing that people with chronic illness need clear frameworks and definitive strategies, not vague options.

About the Composite Case Studies

The patient stories that begin each chapter are composite cases created from patterns observed across hundreds of patient experiences. These narratives combine common challenges, successful strategies, and realistic outcomes to illustrate key points while protecting individual privacy. Any resemblance to specific real persons, living or deceased, is purely coincidental.

These composite cases represent typical scenarios rather than exceptional outcomes. They demonstrate both the challenges and possibilities that exist for people managing the trifecta, showing realistic timelines for improvement, expected setbacks, and the incremental progress that characterizes successful chronic illness management.

The patients in these stories—Sarah, Marcus, Jennifer, Katherine, and others—represent the diversity of people affected by these conditions: different ages, backgrounds, symptom patterns, and life circumstances. Their experiences illustrate that while the fundamental strategies for managing POTS, MCAS, and EDS remain consistent, the application of these strategies must be individualized to fit each person's unique situation.

Why This Book

Traditional medical resources often address POTS, MCAS, and EDS as separate conditions, yet patients frequently experience all three simultaneously. This book provides the first comprehensive guide specifically designed for managing these interconnected conditions as an integrated syndrome rather than isolated disorders.

The strategies presented here emerge from patient experiences, clinical research, and the evolving understanding of how these conditions interact. While medical knowledge about the trifecta continues advancing, the practical management approaches detailed in this guide provide a foundation for thriving with chronic illness regardless of future medical developments.

A Note on Medical Advice

This book provides educational information and practical strategies for managing chronic illness but does not constitute medical advice. All treatment decisions should be made in consultation with qualified healthcare providers who understand your specific medical situation. The goal is to help you become a more informed patient and effective advocate for your own care, not to replace professional medical guidance.

The journey from diagnosis to successful management is rarely linear or quick. This guide provides the roadmap, but you must walk the path at your own pace, adapting strategies to fit your unique circumstances and needs. The destination—a meaningful, fulfilling life alongside chronic illness—is achievable for most people willing to invest in learning effective management strategies.

Your chronic illness story is still being written. This book provides tools to help ensure the chapters ahead are filled with purpose, connection, and hope, even when they include ongoing health challenges. The patients whose composite experiences fill these pages prove that extraordinary lives are possible within the boundaries that chronic illness creates.

Welcome to your comprehensive guide for not just surviving, but thriving with the trifecta.

Chapter 1: How POTS, MCAS, and EDS Interact

Marcus collapsed on his kitchen floor at 6:30 AM, his vision tunneling as his heart hammered against his ribs. The simple act of getting up to make coffee had triggered a cascade of symptoms that left him gasping and confused. His skin flushed red and hot, his joints ached despite minimal movement, and his pulse raced past 140 beats per minute. Three separate medical emergencies were happening in his body simultaneously—yet they shared a single, connected cause.

This scenario plays out daily for thousands of people living with the trifecta of POTS, MCAS, and EDS. These conditions don't just happen to occur together by coincidence. They form an interconnected web of dysfunction that affects every system in the body, from the cellular level to complex physiological processes. Understanding these connections transforms scattered symptoms into a coherent pattern that can be managed effectively.

The medical community has traditionally treated these conditions in isolation, sending patients from specialist to specialist without anyone connecting the dots. Cardiologists address the heart rate irregularities of POTS. Immunologists tackle the allergic reactions of MCAS. Rheumatologists or geneticists handle the joint hypermobility of EDS. Yet the most effective treatment approaches recognize that these conditions share common pathways and influence each other in predictable ways.

The Connective Tissue Connection

Your body's connective tissue serves as the scaffolding that holds everything together. Think of it as the internal framework that supports organs, blood vessels, joints, and skin. In EDS, genetic mutations affect collagen production—the primary protein that makes connective tissue strong and flexible. This single defect creates vulnerabilities throughout your entire system.

Collagen's Critical Role

Collagen makes up about 30% of your body's total protein content. It provides structure to skin, strength to blood vessels, stability to joints, and support to organs. When collagen production is compromised, as it is in EDS, the effects ripple through every system in your body.

Blood vessels become more fragile and stretchy. This creates problems with blood flow regulation, contributing to the orthostatic intolerance seen in POTS. Your blood vessels can't maintain proper tension, making it harder for your cardiovascular system to pump blood effectively against gravity.

Joint stability decreases significantly. Without proper collagen support, joints become hypermobile and prone to injury. This leads to chronic pain, frequent dislocations, and the constant muscle tension that develops as your body tries to compensate for unstable joints.

Skin elasticity changes dramatically. EDS patients often have soft, stretchy skin that bruises easily and heals slowly. This same collagen defect affects internal tissues, making them more susceptible to inflammation and injury.

The Vascular Connection

Blood vessel integrity plays a crucial role in both POTS and MCAS symptoms. When collagen defects weaken blood vessels, several problems develop that connect all three conditions.

Orthostatic intolerance occurs when blood vessels can't maintain proper constriction. Normally, when you stand up, your blood vessels tighten to help pump blood back to your heart. In EDS, weak blood vessels can't perform this function effectively, leading to blood pooling in your legs and abdomen. Your heart compensates by beating faster—hence the tachycardia in POTS.

Mast cell activation increases around damaged blood vessels. Your immune system recognizes the ongoing tissue damage and inflammation caused by weak connective tissue. Mast cells, which are your body's first responders to injury, become hyperactive as they try to address the constant low-level damage occurring throughout your system.

Chronic inflammation develops as your body attempts to repair ongoing tissue damage. This creates a cycle where inflammation damages already weak connective tissue, leading to more inflammation. MCAS symptoms often worsen during periods of increased connective tissue stress.

Autonomic Dysfunction Cascade

Your autonomic nervous system controls all the functions you don't consciously think about—heart rate, blood pressure, digestion, temperature regulation, and breathing.

POTS represents a malfunction in this system, but the dysfunction extends far beyond simple heart rate changes.

The Autonomic Network

Your autonomic nervous system has two main branches that work in balance. The sympathetic system handles "fight or flight" responses, while the parasympathetic system manages "rest and digest" functions. In POTS, this balance becomes disrupted, creating symptoms that affect every organ system.

Cardiovascular symptoms include rapid heart rate, blood pressure fluctuations, and poor circulation. These occur because your autonomic nervous system can't properly regulate blood flow and heart function in response to position changes or physical demands.

Gastrointestinal problems develop because the same nerves that control heart rate also control digestion. Many POTS patients experience nausea, gastroparesis (delayed stomach emptying), and digestive irregularities. These symptoms often trigger MCAS reactions, creating a cycle of autonomic dysfunction and immune activation.

Temperature regulation becomes problematic as your body loses the ability to properly control blood flow to your skin. This leads to feeling cold in warm environments or overheating during minimal activity. Temperature changes often trigger both POTS episodes and MCAS reactions.

The Stress Response Connection

Chronic illness creates ongoing stress on your autonomic nervous system. Your body interprets the constant symptoms and medical challenges as threats, keeping your stress response system activated. This chronic activation worsens all three conditions.

Adrenaline levels remain elevated as your body tries to compensate for poor blood flow and circulation. High adrenaline levels can trigger MCAS reactions and worsen POTS symptoms. You may notice that stressful situations make all your symptoms worse.

Sleep disruption occurs because your autonomic nervous system can't properly transition between waking and sleeping states. Poor sleep worsens POTS symptoms, increases inflammation, and makes MCAS reactions more likely. This creates a cycle where symptoms prevent restorative sleep, and poor sleep worsens symptoms.

Cognitive function declines as your brain struggles with inconsistent blood flow and chronic inflammation. Brain fog, memory problems, and difficulty concentrating are common in all three conditions. These cognitive symptoms often worsen during symptom flares.

Mast Cell Activation as the Inflammatory Bridge

Mast cells are immune system cells that normally protect you from infections and allergens. In MCAS, these cells become hyperactive, releasing inflammatory chemicals in response to triggers that shouldn't cause reactions. This creates the inflammatory bridge that connects POTS and EDS symptoms.

Mast Cell Function and Dysfunction

Healthy mast cells respond to genuine threats like infections or allergens. They release histamine and other chemicals that increase blood flow, create inflammation, and attract other immune cells to fight the threat. In MCAS, this response becomes excessive and inappropriate.

Trigger sensitivity increases dramatically. Normal stimuli like temperature changes, physical pressure, emotions, or certain foods can trigger mast cell activation. These same triggers often worsen POTS symptoms and can cause EDS-related pain and inflammation.

Histamine release affects multiple organ systems simultaneously. Histamine causes blood vessels to dilate and become leaky, leading to fluid shifts that worsen POTS symptoms. It also increases inflammation in joints and connective tissue, worsening EDS-related pain.

Inflammatory cascade develops as activated mast cells release dozens of different chemicals. These chemicals create widespread inflammation that affects every organ system. The inflammation worsens connective tissue damage in EDS and disrupts autonomic function in POTS.

The Inflammation Connection

Chronic inflammation creates a cycle that perpetuates all three conditions. Understanding this cycle helps explain why symptoms often occur in clusters and why treating one condition can improve others.

Connective tissue damage triggers inflammatory responses as your body tries to repair ongoing tissue injury. This inflammation makes connective tissue more fragile and prone to further damage. The cycle continues as new damage triggers more inflammation.

Autonomic dysfunction worsens under inflammatory conditions. Inflammation affects the nerves that control autonomic function, making POTS symptoms more severe and unpredictable. Anti-inflammatory treatments often improve autonomic function.

Mast cell activation increases in response to inflammation. The chemicals released during inflammatory responses can trigger more mast cell activation, creating a feedback loop where inflammation causes more inflammation.

The Symptom Overlap Matrix

Many symptoms occur in all three conditions, making it difficult to determine which condition is causing which symptom. Understanding this overlap helps you and your medical team develop more effective treatment strategies.

Cardiovascular Symptoms

Heart rate irregularities appear in all three conditions but for different reasons. POTS causes rapid heart rate due to autonomic dysfunction. MCAS triggers heart rate changes through histamine release. EDS contributes through poor blood vessel function and blood volume regulation.

Blood pressure fluctuations occur as your cardiovascular system struggles to maintain stable circulation. These changes can trigger symptoms in all three conditions and often occur together during symptom flares.

Chest pain and palpitations develop from multiple causes. POTS creates awareness of heart rate changes. MCAS can cause chest tightness and breathing difficulties. EDS may contribute through chest wall hypermobility and muscle tension.

Gastrointestinal Symptoms

Nausea and vomiting occur in all three conditions through different mechanisms. POTS affects the autonomic nerves controlling digestion. MCAS triggers gastrointestinal reactions through histamine release. EDS can cause structural problems with digestive organs.

Abdominal pain develops from multiple sources. Autonomic dysfunction affects normal digestive processes. Mast cell activation creates inflammation in the digestive tract. Connective tissue weakness can cause organs to shift position abnormally.

Food sensitivities increase as all three conditions affect digestion and immune function. MCAS creates reactions to previously tolerated foods. POTS can worsen with certain dietary triggers. EDS patients often develop gastroparesis and food intolerances.

Neurological Symptoms

Brain fog appears in all three conditions but results from different causes. POTS creates cognitive symptoms through poor brain blood flow. MCAS causes inflammation that affects brain function. EDS may contribute through spinal instability and chronic pain.

Headaches occur frequently and can be triggered by any of the three conditions. POTS headaches often relate to blood flow changes. MCAS headaches typically involve inflammation and histamine release. EDS headaches may result from neck instability or intracranial pressure changes.

Sleep disturbances develop as all three conditions interfere with normal sleep patterns. POTS affects the autonomic control of sleep cycles. MCAS can cause nighttime reactions and temperature regulation problems. EDS contributes through pain and difficulty finding comfortable positions.

Case Studies: Three Detailed Patient Profiles

Real patient stories illustrate how the trifecta presents differently in different people. Each case shows the unique combinations of symptoms and the connections between conditions.

Case Study 1: Emma, Age 24 - The Athletic Decline

Emma was a competitive swimmer throughout high school and college. At 22, she began experiencing episodes of rapid heart rate and dizziness after training sessions. Initially attributed to overtraining, her symptoms gradually worsened and began occurring during daily activities.

Her first major episode happened during a routine medical appointment. Standing up from the examination table, her heart rate jumped from 70 to 150 beats per minute. Her skin flushed red, she felt nauseous, and her vision became blurry. The episode lasted fifteen minutes and left her exhausted for hours.

Emma's diagnostic journey took two years and involved multiple specialists. A cardiologist diagnosed POTS after a tilt table test showed dramatic heart rate increases with position changes. An allergist identified MCAS after Emma experienced severe reactions to foods she'd eaten her whole life. A rheumatologist diagnosed EDS after noting her joint hypermobility and family history of similar symptoms.

The connections became clear when Emma learned that her athletic career had likely masked early EDS symptoms. Years of intense training had built muscle strength that compensated for joint instability. When she reduced her training load, her joints became less stable, triggering inflammation and mast cell activation. The chronic inflammation worsened her autonomic dysfunction, leading to more severe POTS symptoms.

Emma's treatment plan addresses all three conditions simultaneously. She takes a beta-blocker for POTS, antihistamines for MCAS, and follows a modified exercise program that builds stability without triggering symptoms. Her diet eliminates known MCAS triggers while providing adequate sodium and fluids for POTS management.

Case Study 2: David, Age 45 - The Corporate Crash

David worked in high-stress corporate finance for twenty years before his symptoms began. His initial complaints seemed stress-related—fatigue, difficulty concentrating, and frequent headaches. His primary care physician recommended stress management and prescribed antidepressants.

The turning point came during a business trip. David experienced severe abdominal pain, flushing, and rapid heart rate after eating at a restaurant. The emergency department attributed it to food poisoning, but similar episodes continued after he returned home. Simple activities like showering or walking upstairs left him exhausted and symptomatic.

David's wife noticed his joints were unusually flexible and that he bruised easily. She researched his symptoms online and suggested he might have EDS. A geneticist confirmed the diagnosis and referred him to specialists for POTS and MCAS evaluation.

The connections in David's case centered around stress and inflammation. Years of high-stress work had likely kept his immune system in a hyperactive state. When combined with EDS-related tissue fragility, this created conditions for MCAS development. The chronic inflammation and autonomic stress contributed to POTS symptoms that worsened over time.

David's treatment required significant lifestyle modifications. He reduced his work hours and stress levels, which improved all three conditions. His medication regimen includes treatments for each condition, but the most significant improvements came from addressing the underlying stress and inflammation that connected all his symptoms.

Case Study 3: Maria, Age 33 - The New Mother's Mystery

Maria's symptoms began shortly after her second pregnancy. She attributed her fatigue and heart palpitations to sleep deprivation and the stress of caring for two young children. However, her symptoms worsened rather than improved as her baby grew older.

Her symptoms followed a pattern that initially confused her medical team. She would have several good days followed by severe symptom flares that included rapid heart rate, skin reactions, joint pain, and extreme fatigue. These flares seemed to occur randomly and lasted for several days.

Maria's diagnosis came after she started tracking her symptoms and triggers. She noticed that her flares often coincided with hormonal changes, weather patterns, and stress levels. Her medical team eventually diagnosed all three conditions and helped her understand their interconnections.

The pregnancy had likely triggered changes in Maria's immune system and hormones that unmasked her underlying EDS and precipitated MCAS development. The physical stress of pregnancy and childbirth, combined with sleep deprivation and hormonal changes, created conditions for POTS to develop.

Maria's treatment plan accounts for her role as a mother and the practical challenges of managing chronic illness while caring for children. Her family learned to recognize early warning signs of flares and developed strategies to manage household responsibilities during difficult periods.

Interactive Symptom Mapping

Understanding your personal symptom pattern requires systematic observation and tracking. This audio-guided exercise helps you identify the connections between your symptoms and recognize your unique trifecta presentation.

Mapping Your Symptoms

Begin by listing all your symptoms, regardless of which condition you think causes them. Include physical symptoms, cognitive changes, emotional fluctuations, and sleep disturbances. Don't worry about categorizing them initially—just capture everything you experience.

Identify symptom clusters that occur together. Notice which symptoms tend to appear at the same time or in sequence. These clusters often reveal the connections between your conditions. For example, you might notice that rapid heart rate occurs with skin flushing and joint pain, suggesting a connection between POTS, MCAS, and EDS symptoms.

Track symptom timing and triggers. Note when symptoms occur, how long they last, and what might have triggered them. Common triggers include position changes, temperature variations, stress, certain foods, hormonal changes, and weather patterns.

Look for patterns in your symptom intensity. Some people have constant low-level symptoms with periodic flares. Others experience symptom-free periods followed by severe episodes. Understanding your pattern helps predict and manage symptom changes.

Identifying Your Triggers

Environmental triggers affect all three conditions but may have different effects in each person. Temperature changes often trigger POTS symptoms through effects on blood vessel function. The same temperature changes may trigger MCAS reactions and worsen EDS joint pain.

Dietary triggers are particularly important in MCAS but can also affect POTS and EDS symptoms. High-histamine foods may trigger MCAS reactions. High-sodium foods may help POTS symptoms but worsen other conditions. Identifying your specific dietary triggers requires careful tracking and sometimes elimination diets.

Physical triggers include position changes, exercise, and physical stress. These triggers often affect multiple conditions simultaneously. Standing up quickly may trigger POTS symptoms, while the resulting stress response may trigger MCAS reactions.

Emotional triggers affect all three conditions through the autonomic nervous system and stress response pathways. Anxiety, excitement, and stress can trigger symptoms in all three conditions. Learning to manage emotional triggers becomes an important part of treatment.

The Domino Effect

Treating one condition often improves symptoms in the others, creating positive cascades of improvement. Understanding these connections helps you and your medical team prioritize treatments and set realistic expectations.

Treatment Connections

Antihistamines prescribed for MCAS often improve POTS symptoms by reducing inflammation and stabilizing blood vessels. Many patients notice that their heart rate becomes more stable and their exercise tolerance improves when their mast cell activation is well-controlled.

Beta-blockers used for POTS can help MCAS symptoms by reducing the stress response that triggers mast cell activation. Some patients find that their allergic reactions become less severe when their autonomic nervous system is more stable.

Physical therapy for EDS joint stability often improves POTS symptoms by improving circulation and reducing the physical stress that triggers autonomic dysfunction. Better joint stability reduces the energy expenditure required for daily activities, leaving more energy for other functions.

Dietary modifications for MCAS frequently help POTS symptoms by reducing inflammation and improving digestive function. When your digestive system works more efficiently, it places less stress on your autonomic nervous system.

Negative Cascades

Understanding how untreated conditions worsen each other helps explain why early intervention is so important. When one condition is poorly controlled, it creates stress that worsens the others.

Uncontrolled MCAS creates chronic inflammation that damages connective tissue, worsening EDS symptoms. The inflammation also affects autonomic function, making POTS symptoms more severe and unpredictable.

Poorly managed POTS creates chronic stress on your cardiovascular system. This stress can trigger mast cell activation and worsen MCAS symptoms. The poor circulation associated with POTS can also contribute to connective tissue damage.

Untreated EDS creates ongoing tissue damage and inflammation. This chronic inflammation can trigger mast cell activation and worsen autonomic function. The pain and physical limitations of EDS also create emotional stress that affects both POTS and MCAS.

Genetic Factors and Family History

Understanding the genetic aspects of the trifecta helps explain why these conditions occur together and what it means for your family members. While genetics play a role, environmental factors and lifestyle choices also significantly influence symptom development and severity.

Inheritance Patterns

EDS follows known genetic inheritance patterns, with most types inherited in an autosomal dominant manner. This means that if one parent has EDS, each child has a 50% chance of inheriting the genetic mutation. However, having the genetic mutation doesn't guarantee that symptoms will develop or be severe.

POTS and MCAS inheritance patterns are less clear but appear to have genetic components. Many patients report family members with similar symptoms, suggesting genetic predisposition. However, these conditions likely result from multiple genetic and environmental factors working together.

The trifecta combination may occur more frequently in families due to shared genetic vulnerabilities. If you have the genetic predisposition for connective tissue problems, you may be more likely to develop autonomic dysfunction and immune system hyperactivity.

Family Screening and Awareness

Family members should be aware of trifecta symptoms and seek evaluation if they develop similar problems. Early recognition and treatment can prevent severe symptoms and improve long-term outcomes.

Children of parents with trifecta conditions should be monitored for signs of joint hypermobility, autonomic dysfunction, and allergic reactions. Many symptoms can be managed effectively when identified early.

Genetic counseling can help families understand inheritance risks and make informed decisions about family planning. Some forms of EDS have more severe symptoms than others, and genetic testing can provide information about specific risks.

Research Frontiers

Scientific understanding of the trifecta continues to advance, offering hope for better treatments and potentially new therapeutic approaches. Current research focuses on the connections between conditions and developing treatments that address multiple conditions simultaneously.

Recent studies have identified specific genetic mutations that may predispose people to developing multiple conditions within the trifecta. This research may lead to genetic testing that can predict risk and guide preventive interventions.

Inflammatory pathway research is revealing how chronic inflammation connects all three conditions. New anti-inflammatory treatments specifically designed for trifecta patients are being developed and tested.

Autonomic nervous system research is advancing understanding of how connective tissue disorders affect nerve function. This research may lead to new treatments that address the root causes of autonomic dysfunction rather than just managing symptoms.

The connections between POTS, MCAS, and EDS represent more than just medical curiosity—they provide the framework for understanding how your body systems interact and influence each other. This understanding transforms a collection of confusing symptoms into a coherent pattern that can be managed effectively.

Marcus, whose story opened this section, learned to recognize his early warning signs and developed strategies that address all three conditions simultaneously. He now manages his symptoms effectively and rarely experiences the severe episodes that once left him collapsed on his kitchen floor. His success came from understanding the connections between his conditions and working with a medical team that treated him as a whole person rather than a collection of separate symptoms.

Practical Applications

The knowledge you've gained about trifecta connections provides the foundation for developing effective management strategies. Every treatment decision should consider how it might affect all three conditions. Every lifestyle modification should account for the interconnected nature of your symptoms.

Your symptom tracking will be more effective now that you understand the connections between conditions. Look for patterns that cross condition boundaries. Notice how treating one condition affects others. Use this information to guide your treatment decisions and communicate more effectively with your medical team.

The next step in your journey involves understanding the diagnostic process and building the medical team that will help you manage these connected conditions. Armed with knowledge about how POTS, MCAS, and EDS interact, you're better prepared to advocate for appropriate testing and treatment.

The connections between these conditions mean that your treatment plan will be more effective when it addresses all three simultaneously rather than treating each in isolation. This integrated approach requires coordination between multiple specialists and a clear understanding of how treatments for one condition might affect the others.

Key Insights From This Foundation

- Connective tissue defects in EDS create system-wide vulnerabilities that contribute to POTS and MCAS

- Autonomic dysfunction affects every organ system, creating symptoms that interact with immune and connective tissue problems

- Mast cell activation serves as an inflammatory bridge connecting all three conditions

- Symptom overlap makes diagnosis challenging but reveals important treatment opportunities

- Treating one condition often improves others through shared pathways and reduced overall body stress

- Genetic factors contribute to trifecta development but environmental triggers and lifestyle factors significantly influence symptom severity

- Understanding connections between conditions enables more effective treatment planning and symptom management

Chapter 2: Navigating Your Diagnostic Odyssey

The medical chart in Dr. Thompson's hands contained four years of conflicting diagnoses, normal test results, and frustrated notes from specialists who couldn't explain Jennifer's symptoms. "Anxiety disorder," read one entry. "Chronic fatigue syndrome," suggested another. "Functional somatic syndrome," concluded a third. Yet none of these diagnoses explained why Jennifer's heart rate jumped to 160 beats per minute when she stood up, why she developed hives after eating foods she'd enjoyed her whole life, or why her joints dislocated during routine activities.

Jennifer's experience represents the typical diagnostic journey for trifecta patients—a frustrating maze of appointments, tests, and dismissals that averages five to ten years from symptom onset to accurate diagnosis. The delay isn't just inconvenient; it's harmful. Each year without proper treatment allows symptoms to worsen, quality of life to decline, and secondary complications to develop.

This extended timeline occurs because the trifecta challenges traditional medical thinking. Most physicians are trained to look for single causes of symptoms, but POTS, MCAS, and EDS create overlapping symptom patterns that don't fit neatly into conventional diagnostic categories. Symptoms that should point to cardiac problems also suggest immune dysfunction. Signs that indicate joint disorders also point to neurological issues.

The good news is that diagnostic methods are improving as awareness of these conditions grows. More physicians recognize the trifecta pattern, better testing protocols are being developed, and patient advocacy is driving changes in medical education. Understanding the diagnostic process helps you become an active participant in your care rather than a passive recipient of medical opinions.

The Diagnostic Timeline

The journey from symptoms to diagnosis follows predictable patterns that can help you understand where you are in the process and what to expect next. Recognizing these patterns also helps you avoid common pitfalls that can delay accurate diagnosis.

Phase One: Symptom Onset and Initial Confusion

Most trifecta symptoms begin gradually, often during periods of physical or emotional stress. Pregnancy, illness, surgery, or major life changes frequently trigger the onset of symptoms in people with genetic predisposition. This timing often leads to initial misattribution of symptoms to temporary stressors.

Early symptoms are often dismissed as normal responses to stress, aging, or lifestyle factors. Fatigue gets attributed to busy schedules. Heart palpitations are blamed on anxiety. Joint pain is dismissed as normal wear and tear. This dismissal can continue for months or years, delaying the start of proper evaluation.

Symptom progression typically follows a pattern of gradual worsening with intermittent flares. Patients often report that symptoms were manageable initially but gradually became more frequent and severe. The episodic nature of many trifecta symptoms can make them difficult to capture during medical appointments.

Primary care physicians often provide the first medical evaluation, but most haven't received training in recognizing trifecta conditions. This isn't a criticism of primary care—these are complex, relatively rare conditions that weren't well-understood until recently. However, it does mean that initial medical evaluations often miss important clues.

Phase Two: Specialist Referrals and Fragmented Care

When primary care physicians can't explain symptoms, they typically refer patients to specialists based on the most prominent symptom. This approach, while logical, often leads to fragmented care that misses the connections between symptoms.

Cardiology referrals usually occur when heart rate irregularities or chest pain become prominent. Cardiologists may perform excellent cardiac evaluations but often miss the orthostatic component that would suggest POTS. Standard cardiac tests like echocardiograms and stress tests are typically normal in POTS patients, leading to discharge without diagnosis.

Immunology or allergy referrals happen when patients develop new food sensitivities or environmental reactions. However, many allergists aren't familiar with MCAS, which doesn't show up on standard allergy tests. Patients may be told they don't have allergies despite having clear reactions to multiple triggers.

Rheumatology referrals often result from joint pain and hypermobility complaints. While rheumatologists are more likely to recognize EDS than other specialists, many focus on ruling out inflammatory arthritis rather than evaluating for hypermobility disorders.

Neurology referrals occur when patients report headaches, cognitive symptoms, or dizziness. Neurologists may perform extensive testing to rule out serious conditions but often miss the autonomic component of symptoms that would suggest POTS.

Phase Three: Pattern Recognition and Accurate Diagnosis

Accurate diagnosis usually occurs when a physician recognizes the pattern of symptoms across multiple organ systems. This recognition often comes from physicians who specialize in trifecta conditions or who have seen enough patients to recognize the pattern.

The "aha moment" frequently occurs when someone— whether a physician, patient, or family member—connects the dots between seemingly unrelated symptoms. Many patients report that they suspected the diagnosis before their physicians did, often after researching symptoms online or connecting with patient communities.

Confirmation testing validates the clinical suspicion but doesn't always provide definitive answers. POTS diagnosis relies on demonstrating heart rate increases with position changes. MCAS diagnosis requires elevated markers during reactions or improvement with antihistamines. EDS diagnosis often depends on clinical criteria rather than specific tests.

The timeline from suspicion to confirmation can vary significantly. Some patients receive all three diagnoses during a single evaluation with a knowledgeable physician. Others may receive diagnoses sequentially over months or years as different specialists evaluate different symptom patterns.

Essential Tests and What They Mean

Understanding the testing process helps you prepare for evaluations and interpret results. Each condition has specific tests that aid in diagnosis, but the interpretation of these tests requires clinical expertise and understanding of the patient's complete symptom picture.

POTS Testing Protocols

The tilt table test remains the gold standard for POTS diagnosis, but it's not always necessary or available. This test involves lying on a table that tilts upright while monitoring heart rate and blood pressure. A heart rate increase of 30 beats per minute or more (40 in adolescents) within 10 minutes of tilting suggests POTS.

Active standing tests can be performed in any medical office and provide similar information to tilt table tests. The patient lies down for several minutes, then stands while heart rate and blood pressure are monitored. This test is more practical for routine use and can be repeated to monitor treatment response.

Holter monitoring captures heart rate patterns over 24-48 hours during normal activities. This can reveal patterns of heart rate variability and help identify triggers for symptoms. Some patients have normal heart rates during medical visits but significant abnormalities during daily activities.

Autonomic function testing evaluates the broader autonomic nervous system beyond just heart rate responses. These tests can identify patterns of dysfunction that help guide treatment decisions. However, these specialized tests are only available at certain medical centers.

Blood volume studies may reveal the reduced blood volume that contributes to POTS symptoms in some patients. This information can guide treatment decisions about fluid and salt intake or medications that affect blood volume.

MCAS Diagnostic Approaches

MCAS diagnosis remains challenging because symptoms can be intermittent and testing must often be performed during active reactions. This creates practical difficulties in capturing the biochemical evidence needed for definitive diagnosis.

Tryptase levels should be measured both at baseline and during symptom flares when possible. Elevated tryptase during reactions supports MCAS diagnosis, but normal levels don't rule it out. Some patients have MCAS with consistently normal tryptase levels.

Histamine metabolites in urine can provide evidence of mast cell activation, but the timing of collection is critical. Samples must be collected within a few hours of symptom onset to capture elevated levels. Many patients have normal results despite having clear MCAS symptoms.

Prostaglandin metabolites offer another marker of mast cell activation. Like histamine metabolites, timing is critical for capturing elevated levels. Some patients have elevated prostaglandin metabolites when other markers are normal.

Response to antihistamine treatment often provides the strongest evidence for MCAS diagnosis. Patients who experience significant symptom improvement with H1 and H2 antihistamines likely have MCAS, even if biochemical markers are normal.

Bone marrow biopsy is rarely needed for MCAS diagnosis but may be performed to rule out mastocytosis if other markers are consistently elevated. This invasive test is only necessary in specific clinical situations.

EDS Evaluation Methods

EDS diagnosis relies primarily on clinical evaluation rather than specific laboratory tests. Most types of EDS are diagnosed based on physical examination findings and family history rather than genetic testing.

The Beighton score assesses joint hypermobility using a nine-point system. Patients are evaluated for their ability to perform specific movements that indicate joint hypermobility. However, joint hypermobility alone doesn't diagnose EDS—other clinical criteria must also be met.

Skin examination evaluates for the soft, stretchy, fragile skin characteristic of many EDS types. Physicians look for unusual scarring patterns, easy bruising, and abnormal skin texture. These findings, combined with joint hypermobility, support EDS diagnosis.

Family history assessment is crucial because most EDS types are inherited. Patients are asked about family members with similar symptoms, joint problems, or unusual medical histories. A strong family history of connective tissue problems supports EDS diagnosis.

Genetic testing is available for some EDS types but isn't always necessary or conclusive. Classical EDS and vascular EDS have specific genetic tests, but hypermobile EDS (the most common type) doesn't have a genetic test available yet.

Specialized testing may be needed for certain EDS types. Vascular EDS requires specific genetic testing because of the serious complications associated with this type. Other specialized tests might be needed based on specific symptoms or family history.

Specialist Mapping

Understanding which specialists handle which aspects of trifecta care helps you build an effective medical team and know what to expect from each appointment. Each specialist brings different expertise and perspectives to your care.

Cardiology and POTS Management

Cardiologists with autonomic expertise provide the most effective POTS care. However, not all cardiologists are familiar with POTS, and some may focus on ruling out structural heart disease rather than evaluating autonomic function. Electrophysiologists, who specialize in heart rhythm disorders, are often more familiar with POTS than general cardiologists.

Cardiac testing typically includes electrocardiograms, echocardiograms, and exercise testing to rule out structural heart disease. These tests are usually normal in POTS patients, but they're important for excluding other conditions that can cause similar symptoms.

Medication management for POTS often involves medications that affect heart rate, blood pressure, or blood volume. Cardiologists are comfortable prescribing and monitoring these medications and adjusting dosages based on response and side effects.

Exercise prescription from cardiology may include specific heart rate targets and activity recommendations. Some cardiologists work with exercise physiologists to develop structured exercise programs for POTS patients.

Immunology and MCAS Care

Immunologists or allergists with MCAS expertise provide the most effective care for this condition. However, MCAS is not widely recognized among allergists, and many focus on traditional allergic conditions rather than mast cell disorders.

Allergy testing typically shows normal results in MCAS patients, which can be confusing for both patients and physicians. MCAS reactions don't involve traditional allergic mechanisms, so standard allergy tests don't identify MCAS triggers.

Medication management for MCAS often involves multiple antihistamines and mast cell stabilizers. Physicians familiar with MCAS understand the need for combination therapy and higher doses than typically used for allergies.

Trigger identification requires working with physicians who understand MCAS trigger patterns. These physicians can help identify environmental, dietary, and lifestyle triggers that might not be obvious to general allergists.

Genetics and EDS Evaluation

Medical geneticists provide the most expert EDS evaluation and can distinguish between different EDS types. They're trained to recognize the subtle differences between EDS types and can provide appropriate genetic counseling.

Clinical evaluation by geneticists includes detailed physical examination, family history assessment, and evaluation of symptoms across multiple organ systems. They're trained to recognize the patterns that distinguish EDS from other connective tissue disorders.

Genetic testing recommendations come from geneticists who understand which EDS types have available tests and which patients would benefit from testing. They can also provide information about inheritance patterns and family planning considerations.

Coordination with other specialists is often provided by geneticists who understand how EDS affects multiple organ systems. They can help coordinate care and ensure that all physicians understand the implications of EDS for their specialty area.

Physical Medicine and Rehabilitation

Physical medicine and rehabilitation physicians (physiatrists) understand the functional implications of chronic conditions and can provide coordination between multiple specialists and can provide coordination between multiple specialists. They focus on optimizing function and quality of life rather than just treating diseases, making them valuable team members for trifecta patients.

Functional assessment by physiatrists evaluates how symptoms affect daily activities, work performance, and overall functioning. This perspective complements the disease-focused approaches of other specialists and helps guide practical treatment decisions.

Exercise and rehabilitation programs from physiatrists are designed specifically for patients with chronic conditions.

They understand how to balance activity with symptom management and can develop programs that improve function without triggering symptom flares.

Pain management approaches from physiatrists often include non-pharmacological options like physical therapy, occupational therapy, and adaptive equipment. They understand chronic pain patterns and can develop multimodal treatment approaches.

Disability evaluation and documentation may be provided by physiatrists who understand the functional limitations created by chronic conditions. This expertise can be valuable for workplace accommodations or disability applications.

Insurance Navigation

Insurance coverage for trifecta evaluation and treatment can be challenging because these conditions are not widely recognized by insurance companies. Understanding insurance processes helps you advocate for necessary care and avoid denials that could delay treatment.

Prior Authorization Strategies

Specialist referrals often require prior authorization, especially for multiple specialists or repeated visits. Understanding your insurance's referral process helps you plan ahead and avoid delays in accessing care.

Testing authorization may be needed for specialized tests like tilt table tests or genetic testing. Working with your physician's office to provide appropriate documentation and justification can improve the chances of approval.

Medication coverage varies significantly between insurance plans, and many trifecta medications are expensive. Understanding your plan's formulary and prior authorization requirements helps you and your physicians choose covered medications when possible.

Appeal processes become important when initial requests are denied. Most insurance companies have formal appeal procedures that allow you to challenge coverage denials with additional documentation and physician support.

Documentation Requirements

Medical necessity documentation should clearly explain why specific tests, treatments, or specialist visits are needed for your conditions. Working with physicians who understand insurance requirements can improve approval rates.

Symptom documentation through detailed records of symptoms, triggers, and treatment responses provides evidence of medical necessity. This documentation becomes particularly important for expensive treatments or repeated specialist visits.

Functional impact documentation shows how symptoms affect your ability to work, perform daily activities, and maintain quality of life. This information supports requests for accommodations or treatments that improve function.

Treatment failure documentation provides evidence that simpler or less expensive treatments have been tried without success. This progressive approach often satisfies insurance requirements for more expensive or specialized treatments.

Preparing for Appointments

Effective appointment preparation maximizes the value of limited time with specialists and increases the likelihood of accurate diagnosis and appropriate treatment recommendations.

The Golden Hour Consultation Strategy

Most specialist appointments last 30-60 minutes, making efficient use of this time crucial for successful outcomes. The "Golden Hour" strategy involves preparing specific information and questions that help physicians understand your condition quickly and accurately.

Symptom timeline preparation involves creating a clear chronological account of when symptoms began, how they've progressed, and what treatments you've tried. This timeline helps physicians understand the pattern and evolution of your condition.

Trigger identification before appointments helps physicians understand what makes your symptoms better or worse. Bringing specific examples of triggers and responses provides valuable diagnostic information.

Treatment response documentation shows physicians what you've tried and how you've responded. This information prevents repeating ineffective treatments and guides selection of new approaches.

Family history preparation includes information about relatives with similar symptoms or related conditions. This information is particularly important for EDS evaluation but can be relevant for all three conditions.

Medical Records Organization

Digital organization systems allow you to access and share medical information efficiently. Many patients maintain electronic files with test results, physician notes, and treatment records that can be easily shared between providers.

Physical filing systems remain important because not all medical records are available electronically. Organizing paper records by date and provider helps you locate information quickly during appointments.

Test result summaries provide physicians with key information without requiring them to review extensive medical records. Creating simple summaries of important test results saves time during appointments.

Medication lists should include current medications with dosages, previous medications with reasons for discontinuation, and known drug allergies or intolerances. This information is essential for safe prescribing decisions.

Advocating Through Dismissal

Unfortunately, many trifecta patients encounter dismissive attitudes from medical providers who aren't familiar with these conditions. Developing advocacy skills helps you navigate these difficult interactions and continue pursuing appropriate care.

Recognition of Dismissive Patterns

Psychological attribution occurs when physicians suggest that physical symptoms are primarily psychological without adequate evaluation for medical causes. While psychological factors can affect chronic illness, dismissing symptoms as "just anxiety" or "just stress" prevents appropriate medical evaluation.

Minimization responses include physicians who acknowledge symptoms but suggest they're not serious enough to warrant evaluation or treatment. Comments like "everyone gets tired" or "joint pain is normal as you age" minimize legitimate medical concerns.

Gender bias affects many chronic illness patients, particularly women, who are more likely to have symptoms attributed to psychological causes or hormonal changes. Being aware of this bias helps you advocate more effectively for appropriate evaluation.

Age bias can affect both young and older patients. Young patients may be told they're "too young" to have serious medical problems, while older patients may have symptoms attributed to normal aging rather than treatable conditions.

Effective Response Strategies

Direct communication about your symptoms focuses on specific, measurable changes rather than subjective descriptions. Instead of saying "I'm tired all the time," say "My heart rate goes from 70 to 140 when I stand up, and I can only walk two blocks before becoming exhausted."

Documentation requests help ensure that dismissive responses are recorded in your medical record. Asking physicians to document their reasoning for not pursuing evaluation creates accountability and provides evidence if you need to seek care elsewhere.

Second opinion requests are reasonable when physicians can't explain your symptoms or when you feel your concerns aren't being addressed adequately. Most physicians should be willing to provide referrals for second opinions if they can't help you.

Patient rights advocacy involves understanding your rights to medical care and informed consent. You have the right to receive explanations for medical decisions and to seek alternative opinions if you're not satisfied with your care.

Telemedicine Optimization

Telemedicine has become increasingly important for trifecta patients, especially those in rural areas or with limited mobility. Optimizing virtual appointments helps you receive quality care regardless of geographic limitations.

Technology Preparation

Connection testing before appointments prevents technical difficulties that can disrupt consultations. Testing your internet connection, camera, and microphone ensures smooth communication with your physician.

Documentation preparation for virtual visits includes having relevant medical records, test results, and medication lists readily available on your computer or device. This preparation helps maintain efficiency during virtual consultations.

Physical examination limitations in telemedicine require creative solutions. Some physical findings can be demonstrated virtually, while others may require in-person evaluation or coordination with local providers.

Environmental optimization for virtual visits includes choosing a quiet, well-lit space where you can speak privately with your physician. Good lighting and minimal background noise improve communication quality.

Maximizing Virtual Care Effectiveness

Symptom demonstration during virtual visits can help physicians understand your symptoms better. For example, you might demonstrate joint hypermobility or show skin changes that are relevant to your diagnosis.

Real-time symptom capture becomes possible during virtual visits if you experience symptoms during the appointment. This can provide valuable diagnostic information that might not be captured during in-person visits.

Family member participation in virtual visits can be easier than coordinating in-person visits. Having family members available to provide additional history or support can improve the quality of virtual consultations.

Follow-up planning for virtual visits should include clear instructions for when in-person evaluation might be needed and how to contact the physician's office with questions or concerns.

Second Opinion Strategies

Seeking second opinions can be valuable for confirming diagnoses, exploring additional treatment options, or gaining access to specialists with more expertise in trifecta conditions.

Timing Second Opinions

Diagnostic uncertainty warrants second opinions when physicians can't explain your symptoms or when you have concerns about the accuracy of your diagnosis. Getting second opinions earlier rather than later can prevent delays in appropriate treatment.

Treatment failure situations may benefit from second opinions when current treatments aren't providing adequate symptom relief or when you're experiencing significant side effects from medications.

Complex cases involving multiple conditions often benefit from evaluation by physicians who specialize in managing complex medical problems or who have specific expertise in trifecta conditions.

Major treatment decisions like surgery or starting high-risk medications may warrant second opinions to ensure you're making informed decisions about your care.

Selecting Second Opinion Providers

Specialist expertise should guide selection of second opinion providers. Look for physicians who specialize in your specific conditions rather than general practitioners who may not have relevant expertise.

Academic medical centers often have physicians with specialized expertise in rare or complex conditions. These centers may have more experience with trifecta conditions than community physicians.

Patient referrals from support groups or online communities can provide valuable information about physicians who are knowledgeable about trifecta conditions and who provide compassionate care.

Geographic considerations may require traveling for second opinions, but many specialists offer telemedicine consultations that can provide expert opinions without travel requirements.

Jennifer's diagnostic journey, which began this section, eventually led to accurate diagnosis and effective treatment. She found a physician who recognized the trifecta pattern and coordinated appropriate testing and treatment. Her experience transformed from frustration and confusion to understanding and hope.

The diagnostic process for trifecta conditions continues to improve as awareness grows and testing methods advance. Patients who understand the process and advocate effectively for themselves are more likely to receive timely, accurate diagnoses that lead to effective treatment.

Your diagnostic journey may follow a different timeline than Jennifer's, but understanding the process helps you navigate the medical system more effectively. You become an active participant in your care rather than a passive recipient of medical opinions. This partnership with your medical team creates the foundation for successful long-term management of your conditions.

Foundations for Success

The diagnostic phase establishes the foundation for everything that follows in your trifecta journey. Accurate diagnosis provides the framework for understanding your symptoms, selecting appropriate treatments, and building realistic expectations for improvement.

The relationships you build with physicians during the diagnostic process often become long-term partnerships in managing your conditions. Choosing physicians who understand trifecta conditions and who communicate effectively with you creates the support system you'll need for ongoing care.

The knowledge you gain about your specific presentation of these conditions guides all future treatment decisions. Understanding which symptoms belong to which conditions, what your triggers are, and how your conditions interact helps you make informed decisions about treatment options.

Key Learning Points From This Experience

- The diagnostic timeline averages 5-10 years but can be shortened through effective advocacy and appropriate specialist selection

- Each condition has specific testing protocols, but diagnosis often relies more on clinical patterns than test results

- Different specialists provide different perspectives and expertise that contribute to comprehensive care

- Insurance navigation requires understanding authorization processes and documentation requirements

- Effective appointment preparation maximizes limited time with specialists and improves diagnostic accuracy

- Dismissive medical encounters can be navigated through direct communication and appropriate advocacy

- Telemedicine provides access to specialized care regardless of geographic limitations

- Second opinions offer valuable opportunities to confirm diagnoses and explore treatment options

Chapter 3: Assembling Your Dream Team

The conference room at Metropolitan Medical Center buzzed with energy as six different specialists gathered around a table to discuss Rebecca's care. Her cardiologist pulled up her latest tilt table test results. Her immunologist shared data from her recent mast cell activation markers. Her geneticist reviewed her family history and EDS evaluation. For the first time in three years of medical appointments, Rebecca felt like she was being treated as a complete person rather than a collection of separate symptoms.

This multidisciplinary approach represents the gold standard for trifecta care, though it's not always available or necessary for every patient. The ideal medical team coordinates care across specialties, communicates effectively about treatment plans, and provides consistent, evidence-based management that addresses all three conditions simultaneously.

Building such a team requires strategy, patience, and often compromise. Perfect specialists may not exist in your geographic area. Insurance may limit your choices. Some physicians may be excellent clinicians but poor communicators. Your challenge is to assemble the best possible team given your specific circumstances and resources.

The process begins with understanding what each team member should contribute and how the pieces fit together. It continues with research to identify qualified providers and evaluation to determine who works best with your needs and communication style. Finally, it requires ongoing maintenance to ensure that team members continue to coordinate effectively as your needs change over time.

The Ideal Medical Team Structure

Effective trifecta care requires coordination between multiple specialties, but the specific structure of your team depends on your symptoms, geographic location, and insurance coverage. Understanding the ideal structure helps you identify gaps in your current care and prioritize additions to your team.

Primary Care Foundation

Your primary care physician serves as the foundation of your medical team, even when specialists manage most of your trifecta care. Primary care physicians handle routine health maintenance, acute illnesses, and coordination between specialists. They're often the first point of contact for new symptoms or urgent concerns.

Choosing primary care physicians who understand chronic illness makes a significant difference in your care quality. Physicians who are familiar with trifecta conditions can provide better coordination with specialists and make more informed decisions about routine care issues that might affect your chronic conditions.

Communication skills become particularly important in primary care physicians because they often serve as interpreters between specialists and patients. They help you understand specialist recommendations, identify potential conflicts between treatments, and make decisions about care priorities.

Chronic illness management skills distinguish excellent primary care physicians from those who primarily focus on acute care. Look for physicians who are comfortable managing complex medication regimens, coordinating specialist care, and addressing the emotional aspects of chronic illness.

Specialist Team Members

Cardiology or electrophysiology provides POTS management in most cases. Cardiologists with autonomic expertise offer the most specialized care, but general cardiologists who are willing to learn about POTS can also provide effective management. Electrophysiologists may be more familiar with POTS than general cardiologists because they routinely deal with heart rhythm disorders.

Immunology or allergy specialists manage MCAS when they're familiar with this condition. However, many allergists focus on traditional allergic diseases and may not be comfortable managing MCAS. Some rheumatologists or hematologists also have experience with mast cell disorders.

Medical genetics provides EDS evaluation and management, particularly for complex cases or when genetic testing is needed. However, many EDS patients receive care from rheumatologists, physical medicine physicians, or other specialists who understand connective tissue disorders.

Physical medicine and rehabilitation (PM&R) physicians offer valuable perspectives on functional improvement and quality of life optimization. They understand how chronic conditions affect daily functioning and can coordinate rehabilitation services.

Gastroenterology becomes important when digestive symptoms are prominent. Many trifecta patients develop gastroparesis, small intestinal bacterial overgrowth (SIBO), or other digestive complications that require specialized management.

Neurology may be needed for patients with headaches, cognitive symptoms, or neurological complications. Some neurologists specialize in autonomic disorders and can provide expertise in POTS management.

Support Service Professionals

Physical therapy plays a crucial role in EDS management and can help with POTS symptoms through conditioning programs. Physical therapists who understand hypermobility disorders provide the most effective care, focusing on joint stability and functional improvement rather than aggressive stretching.

Occupational therapy helps with daily function optimization and energy conservation techniques. Occupational therapists can evaluate your home and work environments and recommend modifications that reduce symptom triggers and improve function.

Mental health professionals who understand chronic illness provide essential support for coping with the emotional challenges of trifecta conditions. Psychologists or counselors with chronic illness expertise can help with anxiety, depression, grief, and adaptation strategies.

Dietitians with experience in medical nutrition therapy can help optimize nutrition for trifecta management. They understand the dietary restrictions and modifications that may be needed for MCAS and can help ensure adequate nutrition despite food limitations.

Pharmacists, particularly those with clinical training, can provide valuable medication management support. They can help identify drug interactions, optimize dosing schedules, and suggest cost-effective alternatives when needed.

Finding Knowledgeable Providers

Locating physicians with trifecta expertise requires research and often creativity. The pool of knowledgeable providers remains limited, but it's growing as awareness of these conditions increases.

Research Strategies

Professional organization directories provide starting points for finding specialists. The Dysautonomia International website maintains lists of physicians who treat POTS. The Mastocytosis Society has provider directories for mast cell disorders. The Ehlers-Danlos Society offers physician recommendations for EDS care.

Academic medical centers often have physicians with specialized expertise in rare or complex conditions. University hospitals may have autonomic labs, genetic clinics, or immunology departments with trifecta experience. These centers may also participate in research studies that could provide access to cutting-edge treatments.

Published research author searches can identify physicians who have published papers about trifecta conditions. Authors of research papers often have clinical expertise in the conditions they study and may be accepting new patients or able to provide referrals.

Medical conference speaker lists include physicians who present at professional meetings about these conditions. Speakers at dysautonomia, immunology, or genetics conferences often have clinical practices focused on these areas.

Patient Community Resources

Online support groups provide valuable provider recommendations from patients who have direct experience with different physicians. However, remember that individual experiences may not reflect overall provider quality, and what works for one patient may not work for another.

Social media platforms host communities where patients share provider recommendations and experiences. Facebook groups, Reddit communities, and Twitter conversations can provide current information about physician availability and quality.

Local support group meetings offer opportunities to connect with other patients in your geographic area who may have recommendations for local providers. Many cities have dysautonomia or chronic illness support groups that meet regularly.

Patient advocacy organizations often maintain informal networks of provider recommendations. Contacting these organizations directly may provide access to provider lists that aren't publicly available.

Referral Networks

Physician-to-physician referrals often provide the highest quality recommendations because physicians understand each other's expertise and practice styles. If you have one good specialist, ask for recommendations for other team members.

Nurse referrals can be valuable because nurses often have direct experience with how physicians interact with patients and manage complex conditions. Nurses in specialty clinics may have insights into which physicians work well together.

Therapy referrals from physical therapists, occupational therapists, or other healthcare providers can identify physicians who understand multidisciplinary care and work well with therapy services.

Pharmacy referrals may identify physicians who are knowledgeable about complex medication regimens or who are willing to work with pharmacists to optimize drug therapy.

Communication Protocols

Effective communication between team members prevents conflicts, reduces medication errors, and ensures that all providers understand your complete medical picture. Establishing clear communication protocols early in team assembly saves time and improves care quality.

Information Sharing Systems

Electronic health records facilitate communication when all providers use the same system, but this isn't always possible. When providers use different systems, you may need to serve as the communication link between team members.

Patient-controlled health records allow you to maintain a complete medical record that you can share with all providers. Several online platforms allow patients to upload and organize medical information that can be shared securely with healthcare providers.

Provider notification systems should include protocols for sharing important information like medication changes, test results, or symptom changes. Establishing these protocols in advance prevents miscommunication during urgent situations.

Regular communication schedules help ensure that team members stay informed about your care. Some patients establish quarterly or biannual communication between key providers to review progress and coordinate care plans.

Coordination Strategies

Care coordinator designation helps ensure that someone takes responsibility for overall care coordination. This might be your primary care physician, a case manager, or even yourself if you're comfortable with the role.

Treatment prioritization becomes important when multiple providers recommend different treatments or when resources are limited. Having clear protocols for making these decisions prevents conflicts and ensures that the most important treatments are prioritized.

Conflict resolution procedures help address disagreements between providers about treatment approaches. Establishing these procedures in advance prevents delays in care when conflicts arise.

Emergency communication protocols ensure that all team members know how to reach each other during urgent situations. These protocols should include after-hours contact information and clear guidelines about when emergency communication is needed.

Provider Interview Questions

Evaluating potential team members requires asking specific questions that reveal their knowledge, experience, and compatibility with your needs. Preparing these questions in advance helps you make informed decisions about provider selection.

Knowledge Assessment Questions

"How many patients with POTS/MCAS/EDS do you currently treat?" provides insight into the provider's experience with these conditions. Higher patient volumes generally indicate more experience, but newer providers who are enthusiastic about learning may also provide excellent care.

"What treatments do you typically recommend for these conditions?" reveals the provider's treatment philosophy and approach. Look for providers who offer evidence-based treatments and who are open to combination approaches when single treatments aren't effective.

"How do you coordinate care with other specialists?" shows whether the provider understands the need for multidisciplinary care and has systems in place for coordination.

"Are you familiar with the latest research in these conditions?" indicates whether the provider stays current with evolving understanding and treatment options.

Communication Style Evaluation

"How do you prefer to communicate with patients between appointments?" reveals the provider's accessibility and communication preferences. Some providers prefer phone calls, others use patient portals, and some communicate primarily through email.

"How do you handle urgent questions or symptoms?" shows the provider's responsiveness to patient needs and availability during crises.

"What role do you see patients playing in their care?" indicates whether the provider supports patient advocacy and shared decision-making.

"How do you explain medical information to patients?" reveals the provider's communication style and ability to translate complex medical concepts into understandable terms.

Practice Management Questions

"What is your typical appointment length?" helps you understand whether the provider allows adequate time for complex discussions and thorough evaluations.

"How far in advance are you scheduling appointments?" indicates availability and accessibility for ongoing care.

"Do you offer telemedicine appointments?" becomes important for ongoing management, especially if you develop mobility limitations or live far from the provider.

"What insurance plans do you accept?" prevents surprises about coverage and out-of-pocket costs.

Red Flags in Medical Care

Recognizing warning signs of inadequate or inappropriate care helps you avoid providers who may not serve your needs effectively. Some red flags indicate lack of knowledge, while others suggest communication or practice management problems.

Knowledge Red Flags

"These conditions are very rare" may indicate that the provider hasn't encountered many patients with trifecta conditions and may not have adequate experience to provide optimal care.

"You're too young to have these problems" shows age bias and lack of understanding that these conditions can affect people of any age.

"All your tests are normal, so nothing is wrong" indicates lack of understanding that many trifecta symptoms occur despite normal standard testing.

"This is just anxiety" without adequate evaluation suggests psychological attribution without ruling out medical causes.

"I don't believe in these conditions" shows fundamental disagreement with established medical knowledge and suggests the provider won't provide appropriate care.

Communication Red Flags

Rushing through appointments without adequate time for questions indicates that the provider may not have sufficient time to address complex conditions appropriately.

Dismissing patient concerns or symptoms suggests poor communication skills and lack of respect for patient experiences.

Unwillingness to coordinate with other providers indicates isolated practice patterns that don't work well for complex conditions requiring multidisciplinary care.

Defensive responses to questions about treatment options or second opinions suggest inflexibility and potential ego issues that interfere with patient care.

Practice Management Red Flags

Frequent cancellations or rescheduling indicates practice management problems that may interfere with consistent care.

Difficulty reaching the office or getting responses to questions suggests poor communication systems that may be problematic during urgent situations.

High staff turnover or frequent personnel changes may indicate practice instability that could affect continuity of care.

Insurance billing problems or unexpected charges suggest practice management issues that could create financial stress.

Building Provider Relationships

Successful long-term relationships with healthcare providers require effort from both patients and providers. Understanding how to build and maintain these relationships improves care quality and satisfaction for everyone involved.

Initial Relationship Building

Preparation for first appointments includes bringing organized medical records, medication lists, and specific questions. This preparation shows respect for the provider's time and demonstrates your commitment to active participation in your care.

Clear communication about expectations helps establish appropriate boundaries and understanding from the beginning. Discuss your goals for treatment, communication preferences, and any specific concerns or limitations you have.

Respect for provider expertise while maintaining patient advocacy creates a balanced relationship where both perspectives are valued. You can ask questions and advocate for your needs while acknowledging the provider's medical training and experience.

Consistency in appointments and communication helps build trust and understanding over time. Regular appointments and consistent communication patterns help providers understand your baseline and recognize changes in your condition.

Long-term Relationship Maintenance

Regular communication about symptoms, treatments, and concerns helps providers understand your progress and adjust treatments as needed. Don't wait for problems to develop before communicating with your providers.

Appreciation for good care strengthens provider relationships and encourages continued excellent care. Simple thank-you notes or positive feedback can make a significant difference in how providers perceive their relationship with you.

Flexibility with appointment scheduling and understanding of provider limitations helps maintain positive relationships even when perfect availability isn't possible.

Advocacy for provider education about your conditions can help improve care not just for you but for other patients with similar conditions. Sharing relevant research articles or patient organization resources can help providers stay current with evolving understanding.

Geographic Challenges

Patients in rural or underserved areas face unique challenges in accessing specialized care for trifecta conditions. Creative solutions and advocacy may be needed to access appropriate care.

Rural Access Solutions

Telemedicine appointments provide access to specialized care regardless of geographic location. Many specialists now offer virtual consultations that can provide expert opinions and ongoing management without travel requirements.

Regional medical centers may have specialists who serve wider geographic areas. These centers often coordinate care with local primary care providers to minimize travel requirements.

Travel planning for specialist appointments may be necessary when local expertise isn't available. Planning multiple appointments during single trips can maximize the value of travel time and expenses.

Local provider education can help improve care quality in underserved areas. Sharing educational materials with local providers or advocating for continuing education programs can improve local expertise over time.

Insurance and Distance Considerations

Out-of-network exceptions may be available when in-network specialists aren't available in your geographic area. Working with insurance companies to document the lack of local expertise can sometimes result in coverage for out-of-network specialists.

Travel expense planning should include consideration of transportation, lodging, and time off work when accessing distant specialists. Some patient organizations offer travel grants or assistance for patients who need to travel for specialized care.

Coordination with local providers helps minimize travel requirements by having local providers handle routine follow-up and monitoring while specialists provide periodic consultation and treatment planning.

Emergency planning becomes particularly important when your specialist team is geographically distant. Having local providers who understand your conditions and can provide urgent care is essential for safety.

Transitioning Providers

Provider transitions occur for many reasons—physicians retire, move, or change practices. Insurance changes may require finding new providers. Your needs may change as your conditions evolve. Planning for these transitions helps maintain continuity of care.

Planned Transitions

Advanced notice of provider departures allows time to plan transitions and ensure continuity of care. Most providers will help facilitate transfers to new physicians when given adequate notice.

Medical record transfers should be initiated as soon as you know about a provider change. Obtaining copies of all relevant medical records ensures continuity when transitioning to new providers.

Medication refills and ongoing treatment needs should be addressed before provider transitions occur. Having adequate medication supplies and clear treatment plans prevents interruptions in care.

Referral assistance from departing providers can help identify appropriate replacement providers who have similar expertise and practice styles.

Emergency Transitions

Sudden provider departures due to illness, practice closure, or other unexpected events require rapid response to maintain care continuity.

Emergency prescription needs may require coordination with other providers or pharmacists when your regular provider is suddenly unavailable.

Medical record access becomes critical during emergency transitions. Having personal copies of important medical records prevents delays in care when provider records aren't immediately accessible.

Temporary care arrangements may be needed while you search for permanent replacement providers. Hospital systems or urgent care centers may provide temporary management while you locate new specialists.

Rebecca's experience with coordinated care, described at the beginning of this section, represents the ideal outcome of careful team assembly. Her specialists communicate regularly, coordinate treatments, and provide consistent, evidence-based care that addresses all aspects of her trifecta conditions. This coordination didn't happen accidentally—it resulted from careful provider selection, clear communication protocols, and ongoing relationship maintenance.

Your team assembly process may look different than Rebecca's, but the principles remain the same. Start with understanding what you need, research available options, evaluate providers carefully, and invest in building strong relationships with your chosen team members.

The effort invested in team assembly pays dividends for years to come. A well-coordinated medical team provides not just better medical care, but also peace of mind that comes from knowing that knowledgeable professionals are working together to support your health and well-being.

The Path Forward

Your medical team forms the foundation for all other aspects of trifecta management. With the right team in place, you can move forward confidently to address symptom management, lifestyle modifications, and long-term planning.

The relationships you build with your medical team become partnerships that evolve as your needs change and as medical understanding advances. These partnerships provide stability and support during difficult periods and celebration during times of improvement.

The coordination skills you develop in assembling your medical team transfer to other aspects of chronic illness management. You become better at advocating for yourself, coordinating complex schedules, and maintaining multiple professional relationships—skills that serve you well beyond healthcare.

Essential Takeaways From Team Building

- Medical team structure should include primary care foundation, relevant specialists, and support service professionals

- Provider research requires multiple strategies including professional directories, patient communities, and referral networks

- Communication protocols between team members prevent conflicts and ensure coordinated care

- Provider evaluation should assess knowledge, communication style, and practice management before committing to care

- Red flags in medical care help identify providers who may not meet your needs effectively

- Long-term provider relationships require ongoing investment and maintenance from both patients and providers

- Geographic challenges can be addressed through telemedicine, travel planning, and local provider education

- Provider transitions require advance planning to maintain continuity of care and treatment effectiveness

Chapter 4: Becoming Your Own Detective

Advanced Symptom Tracking

Lisa's smartphone buzzed at 2:00 PM with her daily symptom check-in notification. Six months ago, this reminder would have annoyed her—another task on an already overwhelming day. Now, she reached for her phone eagerly, knowing that the data she was about to enter would help solve the mystery of her unpredictable symptoms. Her tracking had already revealed that her POTS episodes peaked during the third week of her menstrual cycle, her MCAS reactions worsened on high-pollen days, and her EDS joint pain increased when barometric pressure dropped below 30.10 inches of mercury.

This transformation from frustrated patient to informed detective represents the power of systematic symptom tracking. Most people with chronic illness experience symptoms that seem random and unpredictable. They feel helpless against their bodies' apparent chaos. Yet underneath this apparent randomness lie patterns—connections between triggers and symptoms, relationships between treatments and outcomes, cycles that repeat predictably once you learn to recognize them.

The art of symptom tracking goes far beyond writing "felt bad today" in a diary. It requires understanding what data to collect, how to organize that information effectively, and most importantly, how to recognize the patterns hidden within your daily experiences. This detective work transforms you from a passive victim of chronic illness into an active participant in your care—someone who understands their body's language and can communicate effectively with medical providers.

Advanced tracking systems capture multiple dimensions of your experience simultaneously. You track not just symptoms, but triggers, treatments, environmental factors, sleep quality, stress levels, and countless other variables that influence how you feel. The goal isn't to track everything possible, but to track the right things in ways that reveal actionable patterns.

Multi-Dimensional Tracking Framework

Effective symptom tracking captures the full picture of your experience rather than isolated data points. Think of your symptoms as threads in a complex web—pulling on one thread affects the entire structure. Your tracking system needs to capture these interconnections.

Symptom Documentation Beyond Basic Logging

Symptom intensity scales provide more useful information than simple presence or absence ratings. Use a consistent scale—many people find 1-10 rating systems work well, with clear definitions for each level. For example, level 1 might mean "barely noticeable symptoms that don't affect activities," while level 10 represents "severe symptoms that prevent all normal activities."

Timing patterns reveal crucial information about symptom behavior. Note when symptoms start, how long they last, and when they resolve. Many trifecta symptoms follow predictable patterns—POTS symptoms often worsen in late afternoon, MCAS reactions frequently occur within hours of trigger exposure, and EDS pain may increase during weather changes.

Symptom combinations occur more frequently than isolated symptoms in trifecta patients. Track which symptoms appear together and in what sequence. You might notice that rapid heart rate always precedes skin flushing, or that joint pain increases before digestive symptoms worsen.

Functional impact measurement helps you understand how symptoms affect your daily life beyond just how they feel. Rate your ability to perform work tasks, household activities, social engagements, and self-care routines. This functional tracking often provides more meaningful information than symptom intensity alone.

Trigger Identification Systems

Environmental triggers include weather patterns, air quality, temperature changes, humidity levels, and seasonal factors. Weather tracking apps can provide detailed environmental data that you can correlate with symptom patterns. Many patients discover strong correlations between barometric pressure changes and symptom flares.

Dietary triggers require careful documentation of everything you consume, including foods, beverages, supplements, and medications. Time-stamp your intake and note any symptoms that occur within 4-6 hours. Food trigger identification often takes weeks or months of careful tracking to establish clear patterns.

Physical triggers encompass activity levels, exercise intensity, sleep quality, and physical stress. Track not just what activities you perform, but how you feel before, during, and after physical exertion. This helps identify your optimal activity levels and recognize early warning signs of overexertion.

Emotional triggers include stress levels, mood changes, anxiety, and major life events. Use simple rating scales to track your emotional state throughout the day. Many patients discover strong correlations between emotional stress and physical symptom flares.

Treatment Response Monitoring

Medication effectiveness tracking goes beyond noting whether you took your medications. Rate symptom levels before and after medication doses, document side effects, and track timing of improvements or worsening. This data helps your medical team optimize dosing and timing.

Non-pharmacological intervention tracking includes dietary changes, exercise modifications, stress management techniques, and environmental modifications. Document what you try, when you try it, and how your symptoms respond. This helps identify which interventions provide the most benefit.

Combination therapy effects require tracking how different treatments interact with each other. Some treatments work better together than individually, while others may interfere with each other. Your tracking data can reveal these interactions.

Treatment timing optimization involves tracking when you take medications or perform interventions relative to symptom patterns. You might discover that taking certain medications at different times of day improves effectiveness or reduces side effects.

Technology Tools for Modern Tracking

Digital tracking solutions offer advantages over paper systems—they're portable, searchable, and can generate reports automatically. However, the best tracking system is the one you'll actually use consistently.

Smartphone Apps for Health Tracking

General health apps like MyFitnessPal, Apple Health, or Google Fit provide good starting points for basic tracking. These apps often include symptom tracking features alongside nutrition and activity monitoring. They sync across devices and can share data with healthcare providers.

Specialized chronic illness apps like ArthritisPower, MyRA, or Symple Symptom Tracker are designed specifically for people with chronic conditions. These apps often include features like customizable symptom lists, trigger tracking, and medication reminders.

Customizable tracking apps allow you to create personalized tracking systems that match your specific needs. Apps like Daylio, Mood Meter, or Journey allow extensive customization of tracking categories and rating systems.

Integration capabilities become important if you use multiple health tracking devices or apps. Look for systems that can import data from fitness trackers, smart scales, blood pressure monitors, and other devices you might use.

Wearable Device Integration

Heart rate monitoring through smartwatches or fitness trackers provides objective data about POTS symptoms. Many devices can detect heart rate spikes, irregular rhythms, and patterns that correlate with symptom reports. This objective data often convinces skeptical healthcare providers.

Sleep tracking reveals patterns in sleep quality, duration, and timing that correlate with symptom severity. Poor sleep often predicts worse symptom days, while good sleep may indicate upcoming improvement periods.

Activity monitoring helps you understand your energy expenditure and identify optimal activity levels. Many wearables can track steps, stairs climbed, active minutes, and calories burned. This data helps you pace activities and avoid overexertion.

Stress monitoring through heart rate variability measurements can identify periods of autonomic nervous system stress that may trigger symptoms. Some devices provide real-time stress alerts that allow you to implement coping strategies before symptoms worsen.

Data Export and Analysis Tools

Spreadsheet integration allows you to export tracking data for advanced analysis. Programs like Excel or Google Sheets can create graphs, calculate correlations, and identify trends that might not be obvious in app interfaces.

Cloud storage ensures your tracking data is backed up and accessible from multiple devices. This prevents data loss and allows you to access historical information during medical appointments.

Sharing capabilities with healthcare providers improve communication and care quality. Many apps can generate reports or export data in formats that medical providers can easily review.

Statistical analysis tools can reveal patterns that aren't obvious through casual observation. Simple correlation analysis can identify relationships between triggers and symptoms, while trend analysis can show improvement or worsening over time.

Pattern Recognition Skills Development

Recognizing patterns in your tracking data requires developing new observational skills. Most people need several weeks or months of consistent tracking before patterns become clear.

Identifying Temporal Patterns

Daily cycles often affect trifecta symptoms in predictable ways. POTS symptoms frequently worsen in late afternoon when blood volume is lowest. MCAS reactions may be more common during certain hours when cortisol levels fluctuate. EDS pain might increase during specific times when joint stiffness peaks.

Weekly patterns can reveal connections to work stress, activity schedules, or social commitments. Many people notice that symptoms worsen during weekdays and improve on weekends, suggesting stress-related triggers.

Monthly cycles, particularly in women, strongly influence trifecta symptoms. Hormonal fluctuations affect blood volume, immune function, and pain sensitivity. Tracking symptoms relative to menstrual cycles often reveals predictable patterns that help with treatment timing.

Seasonal variations affect many trifecta patients through changes in weather, allergen exposure, daylight hours, and activity levels. Some patients experience regular winter worsening or spring improvement that helps guide treatment planning.

Correlation Analysis for Patients

Trigger-symptom relationships become apparent through consistent tracking and careful observation. Start by looking for obvious connections—does eating certain foods consistently lead to symptoms? Do weather changes predict symptom flares? Do stressful events precede difficult symptom periods?

Lag time identification helps you understand how long it takes for triggers to affect your symptoms. Food reactions might occur within hours, while stress effects could take days to manifest. Understanding these timing relationships helps you identify triggers more accurately.

Dose-response relationships show how trigger intensity affects symptom severity. Small amounts of trigger exposure might cause mild symptoms, while larger exposures lead to severe reactions. This information helps you make informed decisions about trigger avoidance.

Threshold effects occur when trigger accumulation reaches a critical point before causing symptoms. You might tolerate individual triggers well but experience severe symptoms when multiple triggers occur simultaneously.

Trend Analysis Methods

Baseline establishment requires tracking during stable periods to understand your normal symptom patterns. This baseline helps you recognize when symptoms are truly worse than usual versus just part of your normal fluctuations.

Improvement detection involves recognizing gradual positive changes that might not be obvious day-to-day. Weekly or monthly averages often show improvement trends that daily variation obscures.

Deterioration recognition helps you identify negative trends before they become severe. Early recognition of worsening patterns allows for proactive intervention rather than reactive crisis management.

Plateau identification helps you recognize when treatments have reached their maximum effectiveness and additional interventions might be needed.

The 28-Day Comprehensive Challenge

Establishing accurate baselines requires intensive tracking over a sufficient time period to capture your natural variations. The 28-day protocol provides enough data to identify patterns while remaining manageable for most people.

Week One Foundation Building

Basic tracking setup involves establishing your tracking system and getting comfortable with regular data entry. Focus on consistency rather than perfection during this first week. Choose tracking categories that are most relevant to your symptoms and avoid trying to track everything at once.

Symptom baseline establishment requires rating your symptoms at the same times each day using consistent scales. Morning, afternoon, and evening ratings capture daily fluctuations and help establish your normal patterns.

Trigger documentation begins with obvious environmental and dietary factors. Don't worry about subtle triggers during the first week—focus on clear, identifiable exposures like specific foods, weather changes, or stressful events.

Sleep tracking includes bedtime, wake time, sleep quality ratings, and any sleep disturbances. Sleep significantly affects all trifecta symptoms, making it one of the most important tracking categories.

Week Two Pattern Recognition

Daily review of tracking data helps you start recognizing patterns as they develop. Spend a few minutes each evening reviewing the day's data and looking for connections between triggers and symptoms.

Trigger hypothesis formation involves developing ideas about potential connections you're observing. These early hypotheses guide more focused tracking in later weeks.

Medication timing optimization begins as you notice how your symptoms fluctuate throughout the day. You might discover that taking medications at different times improves effectiveness.

Activity correlation analysis helps you understand how different types and intensities of activity affect your symptoms. This information guides activity planning and pacing strategies.

Week Three Advanced Tracking

Subtle trigger identification becomes possible as you become more observant and your tracking skills improve. Look for less obvious triggers like specific food combinations, emotional patterns, or environmental factors you hadn't considered.

Combination effect documentation involves tracking how multiple triggers or treatments interact with each other. Many patients discover that they can tolerate individual triggers but react strongly to combinations.

Timing relationship analysis helps you understand the lag time between triggers and symptoms. This information improves your ability to identify causes of symptom changes.

Intervention testing allows you to try specific treatments or modifications and track their effects systematically. This controlled approach helps you evaluate intervention effectiveness.

Week Four Data Analysis

Pattern confirmation involves reviewing three weeks of data to identify consistent patterns. Look for relationships that appear repeatedly rather than occasional coincidences.

Baseline adjustment may be needed as you realize your initial assessments weren't accurate. Many people discover that what they thought was normal actually represents mild symptom states.

Treatment optimization recommendations emerge from your data analysis. You might identify optimal medication timing, helpful activity modifications, or trigger avoidance strategies.

Future tracking protocol development involves deciding which tracking categories provide the most useful information for ongoing monitoring. You can streamline your system to focus on the most valuable data points.

Environmental Trigger Mapping

Environmental factors often have stronger effects on trifecta symptoms than patients initially realize. Systematic environmental tracking reveals these connections and helps guide lifestyle modifications.

Weather Pattern Correlations

Barometric pressure changes affect many trifecta patients through effects on blood circulation, joint pressure, and autonomic function. Track pressure readings alongside symptom ratings to identify your sensitivity threshold.

Temperature fluctuations can trigger POTS symptoms through effects on blood vessel function and MCAS reactions through direct mast cell activation. Note both indoor and outdoor temperatures when tracking environmental triggers.

Humidity levels affect respiratory symptoms, skin reactions, and overall comfort. High humidity often worsens symptoms, while very low humidity can also cause problems.

Storm systems combine multiple environmental triggers—pressure changes, humidity fluctuations, temperature swings, and electromagnetic changes. Many patients report feeling worse before storms arrive.

Allergen Exposure Tracking

Pollen counts correlate with MCAS symptoms in many patients, even those without traditional allergies. Local pollen tracking apps provide daily counts that you can correlate with symptom patterns.

Mold exposure often goes unrecognized but can significantly affect both respiratory and systemic symptoms. Pay attention to symptoms in specific locations, especially basements, bathrooms, or areas with water damage.

Chemical sensitivities develop frequently in MCAS patients. Track exposure to cleaning products, perfumes, air fresheners, and industrial chemicals. Even low-level exposures can trigger significant reactions.

Air quality changes affect respiratory symptoms and general well-being. Monitor air quality indices alongside symptom ratings, especially in urban areas or during wildfire seasons.

Stress and Hormonal Influences

Menstrual cycle tracking reveals hormonal influences on all trifecta symptoms. Many women notice predictable symptom patterns related to different phases of their cycles.

Sleep quality correlation shows how poor sleep affects next-day symptoms. This relationship often becomes obvious through tracking but isn't always apparent without systematic documentation.

Emotional stress quantification helps identify relationships between psychological stress and physical symptoms. Use simple 1-10 stress rating scales to track daily stress levels.

Social situation analysis may reveal that certain environments or social interactions consistently affect your symptoms. This information helps guide social planning and energy management.

Medication Response Tracking

Documenting medication effects requires systematic tracking that goes beyond simple compliance monitoring.

Understanding how medications affect your specific symptom patterns guides optimization of drug therapy.

Effectiveness Documentation

Pre-medication baseline measurement involves rating symptom levels before taking medications. This provides clear reference points for evaluating drug effectiveness.

Peak effect timing identification helps determine when medications provide maximum benefit. This information guides timing of daily activities and additional medication doses.

Duration tracking shows how long medication effects last. This information helps determine optimal dosing intervals and identifies when symptoms return.

Dose-response relationships become apparent when you track symptom improvements relative to medication dosages. This information helps your medical team optimize dosing.

Side Effect Monitoring

Immediate side effects occur within hours of medication administration. Track these alongside therapeutic effects to help your medical team balance benefits and risks.

Delayed side effects may take days or weeks to develop. Long-term tracking helps identify side effects that might not be obviously connected to specific medications.

Interaction effects become important when taking multiple medications. Track how different drug combinations affect both therapeutic responses and side effects.

Tolerance development occurs when medications become less effective over time. Tracking helps identify when dose adjustments or alternative treatments might be needed.

Sleep Quality Correlation Analysis

Sleep significantly affects all trifecta symptoms, making sleep tracking one of the most valuable aspects of symptom monitoring. Understanding your sleep patterns helps optimize both sleep quality and symptom management.

Sleep Architecture Documentation

Bedtime consistency affects circadian rhythm regulation, which influences autonomic function. Track both planned and actual bedtimes to identify optimal sleep scheduling.

Sleep onset time measures how quickly you fall asleep. Difficulty falling asleep often correlates with symptom severity and can indicate need for sleep hygiene improvements.

Sleep fragmentation includes the number and duration of nighttime awakenings. Poor sleep continuity often predicts worse next-day symptoms.

Morning symptoms assessment helps identify sleep-related symptom patterns. Many POTS patients wake with symptoms that improve throughout the morning as they hydrate and move around.

Recovery Correlation Tracking

Sleep debt accumulation occurs when you consistently get less sleep than you need. Track cumulative sleep debt alongside symptom severity to identify critical thresholds.

Recovery sleep effectiveness shows how well extra sleep helps you recover from sleep debt. Some patients find that recovery sleep significantly improves symptoms, while others see minimal benefit.

Sleep quality versus quantity analysis helps determine which factor affects your symptoms more strongly. Some patients need specific amounts of sleep, while others benefit more from high-quality sleep regardless of duration.

Nap timing and effects require tracking to optimize daytime rest. Strategic napping can improve symptoms, while poorly timed naps may worsen nighttime sleep.

Sharing Data with Providers

Your tracking data becomes most useful when you can communicate findings effectively to your healthcare team. Proper data presentation helps providers understand your patterns and make informed treatment decisions.

Data Visualization Techniques

Trend graphs show symptom changes over time in ways that are easy for providers to interpret quickly. Most tracking apps can generate these graphs automatically, or you can create them in spreadsheet programs.

Correlation charts help providers understand relationships between triggers and symptoms. Simple scatter plots can show whether specific triggers consistently correlate with symptom changes.

Summary statistics provide overview information about your symptom patterns. Calculate average symptom levels, frequency of severe episodes, and percentages of good versus bad days.

Timeline presentations combine multiple data types to show complex relationships. These might include symptom levels, medication changes, trigger exposures, and intervention attempts on a single timeline.

Appointment Preparation Strategies

Data selection involves choosing the most relevant information for each appointment rather than overwhelming providers with excessive detail. Focus on patterns that relate to treatment decisions.

Key finding summaries highlight the most important discoveries from your tracking. Prepare 2-3 key points that you want to discuss during each appointment.

Question preparation uses your tracking data to generate specific questions about treatment options, medication adjustments, or lifestyle modifications.

Treatment request documentation provides evidence for specific interventions you'd like to try based on your tracking observations.

Jennifer's story, which opened this section, illustrates the transformation that systematic tracking can create. What began as a simple smartphone reminder evolved into a sophisticated understanding of her body's patterns and rhythms. Her tracking data helped her medical team optimize medication timing, identify previously unknown triggers, and develop targeted interventions that significantly improved her quality of life.

The detective work of symptom tracking requires patience, consistency, and analytical thinking. However, the insights you gain provide the foundation for effective symptom management and informed medical decision-making. You transform from someone who experiences unpredictable symptoms into someone who understands their body's language and can predict and prevent many symptom episodes.

The Foundation for Control

Symptom tracking provides the data foundation that supports all other aspects of trifecta management. Understanding your patterns guides dietary choices, exercise planning, stress management, and medication optimization. This knowledge transforms you from a passive patient into an active participant in your care.

The skills you develop through systematic tracking extend beyond health management. You learn to observe carefully, analyze data objectively, and recognize patterns in complex systems. These skills prove useful in many areas of life and contribute to a sense of mastery and control over challenging circumstances.

Moving forward, your tracking data will guide the specific interventions covered in subsequent sections. The patterns you've identified become the roadmap for nutritional optimization, exercise planning, and lifestyle modifications that can significantly improve your symptoms and quality of life.

Essential Learning Points From Detective Work

- Multi-dimensional tracking captures symptom intensity, timing, triggers, and functional impact simultaneously

- Technology tools enhance tracking consistency and provide objective data that supports subjective reports

- Pattern recognition skills develop over time and reveal connections that aren't obvious through casual observation

- The 28-day challenge provides sufficient data to establish baselines and identify reliable patterns

- Environmental trigger mapping reveals hidden connections between external factors and symptom changes

- Medication response tracking guides optimization of drug therapy timing and dosing

- Sleep quality correlation analysis identifies one of the strongest predictors of daily symptom patterns

- Effective data sharing with providers requires preparation, visualization, and focus on treatment-relevant findings

Chapter 5: Nutritional Optimization

Beyond Basic Anti-Inflammatory

Michael stared at his grocery cart in frustration, holding a package of gluten-free bread in one hand and a list of low-histamine foods in the other. His neurologist had recommended a gluten-free diet for his brain fog. His allergist suggested avoiding high-histamine foods for his MCAS. His cardiologist emphasized increased sodium for his POTS. Meanwhile, his family doctor advocated for a Mediterranean diet to reduce inflammation. Four different dietary recommendations from four different specialists—none of whom seemed to consider how these approaches might work together or conflict with each other.

This scenario reflects the confusion many trifecta patients face when trying to optimize their nutrition. Each condition comes with its own dietary recommendations, and these suggestions often seem contradictory. High-sodium foods help POTS but may worsen inflammation. Anti-inflammatory diets include many high-histamine foods that trigger MCAS reactions. Low-histamine protocols eliminate many nutritious foods that support overall health.

The solution lies not in following separate dietary protocols for each condition, but in developing an integrated approach that addresses all three conditions simultaneously. This requires understanding how different foods affect each condition, identifying individual trigger patterns, and creating sustainable eating plans that support overall health while minimizing symptom triggers.

Nutrition for trifecta patients goes beyond basic healthy eating guidelines. You need strategies that account for brain fog affecting meal planning, fatigue limiting cooking energy, joint problems making food preparation difficult, and digestive issues affecting nutrient absorption. The goal is developing an eating pattern that nourishes your body, minimizes symptoms, and fits realistically into your daily life.

The Trifecta Diet Framework

An effective trifecta diet balances the sometimes conflicting nutritional needs of POTS, MCAS, and EDS. This framework provides structure while allowing flexibility for individual preferences and trigger patterns.

Low-Histamine Foundations

Histamine intolerance affects many MCAS patients, making low-histamine eating a cornerstone of trifecta nutrition. However, low-histamine doesn't mean no-histamine—it means finding your individual tolerance level and managing total histamine load throughout the day.

Fresh foods form the foundation of low-histamine eating because histamine levels increase as foods age, ferment, or undergo processing. Fresh meats, poultry, and fish provide protein without significant histamine content. Fresh fruits and vegetables (excluding high-histamine varieties) supply nutrients and fiber.

Histamine liberators trigger mast cell degranulation even if they don't contain histamine themselves. Common liberators include citrus fruits, strawberries, tomatoes, chocolate, and artificial preservatives. Individual tolerance to liberators varies significantly—some patients react strongly while others tolerate them well.

Diamine oxidase (DAO) enzyme supports histamine metabolism and can be taken as a supplement before meals. Some patients find DAO supplementation allows them to tolerate moderate-histamine foods that would otherwise trigger symptoms.

Anti-histamine foods may help stabilize mast cells and reduce overall histamine load. Quercetin-rich foods like onions and apples, vitamin C sources, and omega-3 fatty acids may provide natural antihistamine effects.

Sodium Optimization for POTS

Adequate sodium intake helps expand blood volume and improve circulation in POTS patients. However, sodium needs vary significantly between individuals and may change based on medication use, exercise levels, and climate.

Sodium targets typically range from 3-10 grams daily for POTS patients, significantly higher than general population recommendations. Work with your medical team to determine appropriate sodium levels based on your blood pressure, kidney function, and symptom response.

Natural sodium sources provide minerals alongside sodium and may be better tolerated than processed high-sodium foods. Sea salt, pink Himalayan salt, and electrolyte supplements offer sodium with additional minerals that support cellular function.

Timing considerations affect sodium absorption and effectiveness. Some patients benefit from spreading sodium intake throughout the day, while others find concentrated sodium doses before challenging activities more helpful.

Food-based sodium strategies include adding salt to cooking water for grains and vegetables, using salted nuts and seeds as snacks, and incorporating naturally sodium-rich foods like olives and pickled vegetables (if histamine-tolerant).

Anti-Inflammatory Principles

Chronic inflammation worsens all three trifecta conditions, making anti-inflammatory nutrition a priority. However, many traditional anti-inflammatory foods are high in histamine, requiring careful selection and preparation methods.

Omega-3 fatty acids provide potent anti-inflammatory effects and may help stabilize mast cells. Cold-water fish like salmon and sardines offer the most bioavailable omega-3s, though fish histamine levels increase rapidly with age. Purchase fresh fish and consume quickly, or consider high-quality fish oil supplements.

Antioxidant-rich foods combat oxidative stress that contributes to inflammation and tissue damage. Berries, leafy greens, and colorful vegetables provide antioxidants, though some high-antioxidant foods like aged cheeses and fermented foods may trigger MCAS reactions.

Gut health optimization reduces systemic inflammation through improved digestive function. Prebiotic foods like garlic, onions, and asparagus feed beneficial bacteria, while probiotic foods support microbiome balance (choose fresh, low-histamine options).

Blood sugar stabilization prevents inflammatory spikes that can trigger symptoms. Balanced meals combining protein, healthy fats, and complex carbohydrates help maintain steady glucose levels throughout the day.

Meal Planning and Preparation Strategies

Successful trifecta nutrition requires planning systems that work during both good days and symptom flares. Your meal planning must account for varying energy levels, cognitive function, and physical abilities.

Energy-Smart Meal Planning

Batch cooking during high-energy periods provides ready-made meals for difficult days. Prepare large quantities of safe foods when you feel well, then freeze in individual portions. Focus on simple, nutrient-dense meals that reheat well.

One-pot meals minimize cooking complexity and cleanup requirements. Slow cooker and pressure cooker recipes allow you to prepare nutritious meals with minimal active cooking time. Sheet pan meals require only simple chopping and assembly.

Ingredient prep strategies involve washing, chopping, and portioning ingredients when you have energy. Pre-washed greens, chopped vegetables, and portioned proteins make meal assembly quick and easy during low-energy periods.

Emergency meal planning ensures you always have safe, easy options available. Keep frozen vegetables, canned low-sodium broth, and shelf-stable proteins on hand for quick meal assembly.

Kitchen Adaptations for EDS

Ergonomic tools reduce joint stress during food preparation. Lightweight cookware, ergonomic knives, and electric can openers minimize strain on hypermobile joints. Jar openers and grip-enhancing tools help with containers.

Counter height organization keeps frequently used items within easy reach to avoid overhead reaching that can stress shoulder joints. Store heavy items at waist level rather than in high cabinets.

Sitting preparation options include high stools or portable chairs that allow you to sit while preparing food. Rolling carts bring ingredients and tools to you rather than requiring multiple trips around the kitchen.

Batch preparation techniques minimize repetitive motions that can trigger joint pain. Chop all vegetables at once rather than preparing each meal individually. Use food processors for tasks requiring repetitive cutting or mixing.

Brain Fog Meal Solutions

Visual meal planning systems work better than written lists during cognitive difficulties. Photo meal plans, color-coded ingredients, and visual recipe cards help when reading comprehension is reduced.

Simple recipe formulas provide structure without requiring complex decision-making. Develop templates like "protein + vegetable + safe starch + healthy fat" that can be customized with available ingredients.

Automated shopping systems through grocery pickup or delivery services reduce decision fatigue and ensure you always have safe foods available. Create saved shopping lists for easy reordering.

Meal timing reminders help maintain regular eating patterns that support blood sugar stability and medication effectiveness. Phone alarms or smartwatch notifications can prompt meal times when hunger cues are unreliable.

Supplement Science for Trifecta Support

Strategic supplementation can address nutritional gaps and provide therapeutic benefits for trifecta symptoms. However, supplement selection requires careful consideration of individual needs, potential interactions, and cost-effectiveness.

Evidence-Based Supplement Protocols

Magnesium glycinate supports muscle and nerve function while being well-tolerated by sensitive digestive systems. Magnesium helps with sleep quality, muscle cramping, and may reduce migraine frequency. Start with 200-400mg daily and adjust based on response and bowel tolerance.

Vitamin D3 optimization supports immune function and may help with fatigue and mood symptoms. Many chronic illness patients have insufficient vitamin D levels. Target blood levels of 40-60 ng/mL through supplementation and regular monitoring.

Methylated B vitamins support energy metabolism and nervous system function. MTHFR gene variations affect folate metabolism in some patients, making methylated forms more effective. B12 deficiency is common in POTS patients and may contribute to fatigue and cognitive symptoms.

Coenzyme Q10 supports cellular energy production and may help with fatigue and exercise tolerance. Choose ubiquinol forms for better absorption. Typical doses range from 100-300mg daily, taken with fat-containing meals.

Histamine-Related Supplementation

DAO enzyme supplements help break down dietary histamine and may allow greater food variety in histamine-sensitive patients. Take 1-2 capsules before meals containing moderate-histamine foods. Effectiveness varies significantly between individuals.

Quercetin provides natural antihistamine effects and mast cell stabilization. Choose quercetin with bromelain for enhanced absorption. Typical doses range from 500-1000mg twice daily, taken away from meals.

Vitamin C supports histamine metabolism and provides antioxidant protection. Use buffered forms to minimize stomach irritation. High doses (1000-3000mg daily) may provide antihistamine effects, but start with lower doses and increase gradually.

Natural antihistamines like stinging nettle, butterbur, and bromelain may provide symptom relief with fewer side effects than pharmaceutical antihistamines. However, herbal supplements can interact with medications and may trigger reactions in sensitive individuals.

POTS-Specific Supplements

Electrolyte supplements help maintain blood volume and improve circulation. Choose products with sodium, potassium, and magnesium in appropriate ratios. Avoid products with artificial colors, flavors, or preservatives that may trigger MCAS reactions.

Licorice root supports blood pressure regulation through effects on aldosterone activity. Use deglycyrrhizinated (DGL) forms to avoid blood pressure elevation in sensitive individuals. Monitor blood pressure regularly if using licorice supplements.

Compression stockings, while not a supplement, provide mechanical support for circulation and can significantly improve POTS symptoms. Graduated compression stockings (20-30 mmHg) are most effective for most patients.

Iron supplementation helps if deficiency is present, as iron deficiency can worsen POTS symptoms. However, iron supplements can trigger digestive symptoms and MCAS reactions in some patients. Use chelated forms and take with vitamin C for better absorption.

Hydration and Electrolyte Management

Proper hydration goes far beyond drinking more water. Trifecta patients need strategic fluid and electrolyte replacement that supports blood volume, cellular function, and symptom management.

Advanced Hydration Strategies

Fluid timing affects effectiveness of hydration efforts. Drinking large amounts of plain water can actually worsen symptoms by diluting electrolytes. Instead, consume smaller amounts of electrolyte-containing fluids throughout the day.

Electrolyte ratios matter for optimal hydration. Sodium helps retain fluid, potassium supports cellular function, and magnesium prevents cramping. Commercial electrolyte products often contain inadequate sodium for POTS patients.

Temperature considerations affect tolerance and absorption. Room temperature or slightly warm fluids may be better absorbed than ice-cold drinks. Some patients find that very cold fluids trigger MCAS reactions.

Fluid types influence how well your body retains hydration. Plain water moves through your system quickly, while fluids containing electrolytes, protein, or small amounts of carbohydrates are retained longer.

DIY Electrolyte Solutions

Homemade oral rehydration solutions provide controlled electrolyte content without artificial additives. Mix 1/4 teaspoon salt, 1/4 teaspoon potassium chloride (salt substitute), and 2 tablespoons sugar in 16 ounces of water.

Natural electrolyte sources include coconut water (high potassium), sea salt (balanced minerals), and bone broth (sodium plus protein). These options provide electrolytes alongside other beneficial nutrients.

Flavor customization helps with compliance and taste preferences. Add fresh lemon juice, herbal teas, or small amounts of fruit juice to electrolyte solutions. Avoid artificial flavors and colors that may trigger reactions.

Concentration adjustments allow you to match electrolyte content to your individual needs and tolerance. Start with lower concentrations and increase gradually based on symptom response and medical team guidance.

Food Sensitivity Testing and Interpretation

Understanding your individual food triggers requires systematic testing approaches that go beyond standard allergy testing. Most MCAS reactions don't involve traditional allergic mechanisms, making specialized testing necessary.

Testing Method Evaluation

IgE allergy testing identifies traditional allergic reactions but misses most MCAS triggers. These tests are useful for identifying true food allergies but won't detect histamine intolerance or mast cell activation triggers.

IgG food sensitivity testing remains controversial with mixed research support. Some patients find these tests helpful for identifying problem foods, while others find them unreliable. Results should be interpreted carefully and confirmed through elimination diets.

Elimination diets provide the most reliable method for identifying food triggers in MCAS patients. Remove suspected trigger foods for 2-4 weeks, then reintroduce them one at a time while monitoring symptoms carefully.

Food challenge protocols help confirm suspected triggers identified through elimination diets. Reintroduce foods in controlled amounts while tracking symptoms for several days. Some reactions may be delayed by 12-24 hours.

Interpreting Results Accurately

False positives occur when test results suggest food sensitivities that don't actually cause symptoms. Always confirm test results through elimination and reintroduction before permanently removing foods from your diet.

Threshold effects mean that you may tolerate small amounts of trigger foods but react to larger portions. This dose-response relationship affects how you interpret and apply test results.

Cumulative effects occur when multiple low-level triggers combine to cause symptoms. You might tolerate individual trigger foods but react when consuming several triggering foods in the same day.

Temporal variations affect food tolerance based on stress levels, hormonal cycles, and overall health status. Foods that trigger reactions during flares may be well-tolerated during stable periods.

Restaurant and Social Eating Strategies

Maintaining social connections while managing dietary restrictions requires planning, communication, and flexibility. The goal is participating in social activities without compromising your health or feeling isolated.

Restaurant Navigation Skills

Menu research before dining out helps identify safe options and reduces decision-making stress during social situations. Many restaurants post menus online, allowing you to plan your order in advance. Look for simple preparations like grilled proteins with steamed vegetables that avoid common triggers.

Kitchen communication with restaurant staff requires clear, specific requests about food preparation. Explain that you have medical dietary restrictions rather than preferences. Ask about ingredient lists, cooking methods, and potential cross-contamination with trigger foods.

Safe ordering strategies focus on simple preparations that minimize unknown ingredients. Choose grilled, baked, or steamed foods over sauced or heavily seasoned options. Request dressings and sauces on the side so you can control portions and ingredients.

Backup planning ensures you always have safe options available. Eat a small meal before going out so you're not overly hungry if restaurant options are limited. Carry safe snacks in case nothing at the restaurant works for you.

Social Situation Management

Communication strategies help friends and family understand your dietary needs without making them the focus of social gatherings. Explain your restrictions briefly and suggest restaurants or activities that work for everyone.

Contribution options for gatherings include bringing a dish you can eat that others will enjoy too. This ensures you have safe food available while contributing to the meal. Share recipes for your safe dishes so hosts can accommodate you in the future.

Event planning involvement helps ensure gatherings include options you can enjoy. Offer to help plan menus or suggest restaurants that accommodate dietary restrictions. Most people want to be helpful once they understand your needs.

Graceful declining techniques help you handle situations where safe food isn't available without causing social awkwardness. Thank hosts for invitations while explaining your limitations. Suggest alternative ways to participate in social activities.

Travel Nutrition Planning

Maintaining your dietary requirements while traveling requires advance planning and creative problem-solving. Travel disrupts normal eating patterns and limits access to familiar foods.

Preparation Strategies

Research destination food options before traveling to identify grocery stores, restaurants, and emergency food sources. Look for accommodations with kitchenettes or refrigerators that allow you to store and prepare safe foods.

Packing safe foods for travel includes non-perishable staples, electrolyte supplements, and emergency meals. Airlines allow medical foods in carry-on luggage—pack supplements and special dietary items in labeled containers with documentation if needed.

Documentation preparation includes letters from your medical team explaining your dietary restrictions for airport security and international customs. Carry prescription information for any supplements you travel with.

Emergency food planning ensures you have safe options if travel plans change or local food sources aren't adequate. Pack extra food for potential delays and identify 24-hour grocery stores or pharmacies at your destination.

Maintaining Routines Away From Home

Meal timing consistency helps maintain stable blood sugar and medication effectiveness during travel. Adjust meal times gradually before traveling across time zones to minimize disruption.

Hydration management during travel requires planning for airport security restrictions and varying access to clean water. Bring empty water bottles to fill after security and consider water purification tablets for international travel.

Supplement scheduling may need adjustment for time zone changes and varying meal times. Pack supplements in daily organizers and set phone alarms to maintain consistent timing.

Activity adaptation affects nutritional needs during travel. Increased walking or activity may require additional electrolytes and calories, while sedentary travel days may need reduced portions.

Budget-Conscious Healthy Eating

Specialized diets often seem expensive, but strategic planning can make trifecta nutrition affordable. Focus on nutrient-dense whole foods rather than expensive specialty products.

Cost-Effective Shopping Strategies

Bulk buying of non-perishable staples like rice, quinoa, and frozen vegetables reduces per-serving costs. Buy meat in bulk when on sale and freeze in individual portions. Purchase spices and seasonings in bulk from ethnic markets or online sources.

Seasonal eating reduces costs while providing variety throughout the year. Learn which fruits and vegetables are in season in your area and plan menus around these affordable options. Preserve seasonal produce by freezing or dehydrating for year-round use.

Generic and store brand products often provide the same quality as name brands at lower costs. Compare ingredient lists rather than focusing on brand names. Many store brands are manufactured by the same companies that make name-brand products.

Coupon strategies work especially well for pantry staples and frozen foods that you use regularly. Stack manufacturer coupons with store sales for maximum savings. Use grocery store apps to find digital coupons and track sales.

Affordable Protein Sources

Eggs provide complete protein at low cost and are well-tolerated by most people with food sensitivities. Buy in bulk when on sale and use in various preparations throughout the week.

Legumes offer plant-based protein, fiber, and nutrients at very low cost. Dried beans and lentils are more economical than canned versions. Prepare large batches and freeze portions for quick meal additions.

Less expensive cuts of meat can be just as nutritious as premium cuts when prepared properly. Slow cooking methods make tougher cuts tender and flavorful. Ground meats are typically less expensive than whole cuts.

Canned fish provides omega-3 fatty acids and protein at reasonable cost. Choose varieties packed in water rather than oil to avoid potential trigger ingredients. Buy in bulk when on sale and store in a cool, dry place.

Maximizing Nutrient Value

Frozen vegetables often provide better nutrition than fresh vegetables that have traveled long distances or been stored for extended periods. They're also more affordable and reduce food waste since you use only what you need.

Organ meats provide exceptional nutrient density at low cost but require acquired tastes and special preparation. Liver is particularly rich in B vitamins and iron. Start with small amounts mixed into ground meat dishes.

Bone broth provides minerals, protein, and gelatin that support joint health. Make your own from bones saved from roasted meats or purchased from local butchers. Freeze in ice cube trays for easy portioning.

Nutrient-dense snacks like nuts and seeds provide healthy fats, protein, and minerals. Buy raw nuts and seeds in bulk and store in the freezer to maintain freshness. Roast small batches with sea salt for homemade snacks.

Cooking Adaptations for Physical Limitations

Joint hypermobility, fatigue, and brain fog affect your ability to prepare food safely and efficiently. Kitchen adaptations and modified techniques help you maintain good nutrition despite physical challenges.

Ergonomic Kitchen Setup

Counter height optimization reduces strain on your back and joints during food preparation. Adjust work surfaces to elbow height when possible, or use cutting boards on top of counters to raise the work surface.

Tool selection focuses on lightweight, ergonomic options that reduce joint stress. Electric can openers, lightweight cookware, and ergonomic knives make food preparation easier. Invest in quality tools that reduce effort and strain.

Storage organization keeps frequently used items within easy reach to avoid overhead stretching or bending. Store heavy items at waist level and use pull-out shelves to improve access to deep cabinets.

Seating options during food preparation prevent fatigue and reduce joint stress. Use a high stool or rolling chair that allows you to sit while working at the counter. Take breaks during longer cooking sessions.

Energy-Conserving Techniques

One-pot cooking methods minimize cleanup while providing nutritious meals. Slow cookers, pressure cookers, and sheet pan meals require minimal preparation and monitoring. Prepare ingredients during high-energy periods for quick assembly later.

Batch cooking during good days provides ready-made meals for difficult periods. Double recipes and freeze half for future use. Prepare versatile base ingredients like cooked grains and proteins that can be combined in different ways.

Assembly-style meals require minimal cooking while providing balanced nutrition. Prepare components like cooked proteins, roasted vegetables, and prepared grains that can be quickly combined for complete meals.

Modified techniques reduce physical demands of cooking. Use kitchen shears instead of knives when possible. Break tasks into smaller segments with rest periods. Use pre-cut vegetables when budget allows.

Safety Considerations

Heat safety becomes particularly important when brain fog affects concentration or EDS affects coordination. Use timers for all cooking tasks and consider induction cooktops that don't stay hot after use.

Sharp tool safety requires extra attention when joint hypermobility affects grip strength or coordination. Keep knives sharp (they require less pressure) and use cutting boards with raised edges to prevent slipping.

Lifting limitations from POTS and EDS require modifications for handling heavy pots and pans. Use smaller cooking vessels and fill them after placing on the stove. Ask for help with heavy lifting tasks.

Fall prevention becomes important when POTS affects balance or EDS affects joint stability. Keep floors clear of obstacles, use non-slip mats, and wear supportive shoes in the kitchen.

Emergency Food Planning

Symptom flares can make cooking difficult or impossible, making emergency food planning essential for maintaining nutrition during difficult periods.

Flare Day Food Strategies

Ready-to-eat safe foods should always be available for days when cooking isn't possible. Stock shelf-stable items like nut butters, crackers, canned soups, and frozen meals that meet your dietary requirements.

Minimal preparation meals require only heating or simple assembly. Pre-cooked proteins, steamed vegetable packets, and instant rice provide balanced nutrition with minimal effort. Prepare these options during well periods.

Comfort food modifications create safe versions of foods that provide emotional comfort during difficult times. Develop recipes for safe soups, smoothies, and simple carbohydrates that soothe without triggering symptoms.

Hydration solutions for flare days include pre-mixed electrolyte drinks, herbal teas, and broths that provide fluid and nutrients. Keep these readily available for quick access during symptoms.

Support System Coordination

Family and friend education helps your support network understand how to help during flares. Teach them about your dietary restrictions and show them where you keep emergency foods.

Meal delivery planning for severe flares might include identifying local restaurants that deliver safe foods or arranging for friends to bring appropriate meals. Research delivery options before you need them.

Shopping assistance arrangements help ensure you always have necessary foods available. Ask family members or friends to help with grocery shopping, or set up grocery delivery services.

Emergency contact lists should include restaurants that accommodate your dietary needs, grocery stores with delivery services, and friends who understand your dietary restrictions.

Michael's grocery store frustration, described at the beginning of this section, transformed into confidence as he learned to integrate multiple dietary approaches into a coherent eating plan. He discovered that many foods could serve multiple purposes—bone broth provided sodium for POTS while being low-histamine for MCAS and anti-inflammatory for overall health. His meal planning evolved from trying to follow separate diet protocols to creating an integrated approach that addressed all his conditions simultaneously.

The key to successful trifecta nutrition lies not in perfect adherence to complex rules, but in developing sustainable eating patterns that support your health while fitting into your real life. You learn to balance ideal nutrition recommendations with practical limitations, finding creative solutions that work within your unique circumstances.

Nourishment as Foundation

Nutrition forms the foundation that supports all other aspects of trifecta management. The foods you choose affect energy levels, inflammation markers, symptom frequency, and treatment effectiveness. Good nutrition doesn't cure chronic illness, but it provides the stable foundation that makes everything else work better.

The eating patterns you establish now will serve you for years to come. Investing time in learning your individual food triggers, developing cooking skills, and creating sustainable meal planning systems pays dividends in improved symptoms and quality of life.

Moving forward, the nutritional foundation you've built supports the exercise and activity modifications covered in the next section. Good nutrition provides the energy for safe movement while preventing the blood sugar fluctuations and inflammatory responses that can interfere with exercise tolerance.

Core Principles From Nutritional Optimization

- Trifecta nutrition requires integrating low-histamine, adequate-sodium, and anti-inflammatory principles into cohesive eating plans

- Meal planning and preparation strategies must account for varying energy levels, cognitive function, and physical abilities

- Evidence-based supplementation can address nutritional gaps and provide therapeutic benefits for specific symptoms

- Hydration and electrolyte management goes far beyond drinking more water and requires strategic timing and composition

- Food sensitivity testing provides starting points but must be confirmed through systematic elimination and reintroduction protocols

- Social eating and travel require advance planning and communication strategies that maintain both nutrition and relationships

- Budget-conscious approaches focus on nutrient-dense whole foods rather than expensive specialty products

- Kitchen adaptations and cooking modifications help maintain good nutrition despite physical limitations

Chapter 6: Movement as Medicine

Exercise Adaptation Strategies

The physical therapist watched in amazement as Janet demonstrated her range of motion. Her shoulders rotated far beyond normal limits, her fingers bent backward to touch her forearms, and her knees hyperextended dramatically when she stood up. "That's incredible flexibility," the therapist commented. "You must be a dancer or gymnast." Janet laughed bitterly. "I wish it were a talent. Actually, this hypermobility is part of why I'm here. Every time I exercise, my joints dislocate, my heart rate goes crazy, and I end up in more pain than when I started."

Janet's experience reflects the complex relationship between exercise and trifecta conditions. Traditional fitness advice doesn't work for people whose joints move too far, whose heart rates spike unpredictably, and whose immune systems react to physical stress. Yet movement remains medicine—when done correctly, exercise improves circulation, reduces inflammation, strengthens supportive muscles, and boosts mood and energy levels.

The challenge lies in finding the sweet spot between beneficial movement and symptom triggers. Too little activity leads to deconditioning, muscle weakness, and worsening symptoms. Too much activity or the wrong types of movement can trigger POTS episodes, MCAS reactions, and joint injuries. Success requires understanding how your body responds to different types of movement and developing personalized exercise protocols that provide benefits without harm.

This personalized approach means abandoning conventional fitness wisdom and learning to listen to your body's unique signals. Heart rate zones designed for healthy athletes don't apply when your autonomic nervous system malfunctions. Flexibility training meant to increase range of motion can be dangerous when your joints already move too far. High-intensity workouts that work for others might trigger severe symptom flares that take days to recover from.

Exercise Physiology for Hypermobility

Understanding how hypermobile joints respond to exercise helps you choose activities that build strength and stability rather than increasing joint vulnerability. The goal shifts from increasing flexibility to creating muscular control around unstable joints.

Joint Stability Versus Mobility

Hypermobile joints lack adequate passive restraints from ligaments and joint capsules, making them dependent on muscular control for stability. Traditional stretching can worsen hypermobility by further loosening already loose structures. Instead, focus on strengthening the muscles that provide dynamic stability around joints.

Proprioception training becomes crucial for people with hypermobile joints because position sense is often impaired. Your brain may not accurately perceive where your joints are in space, leading to poor movement patterns and increased injury risk. Balance exercises, single-leg stands, and closed-chain movements improve proprioceptive awareness.

End-range strengthening targets the muscle lengths where hypermobile joints are most vulnerable. Traditional strength training often focuses on mid-range movements, but hypermobile joints need stability at the extreme ranges of motion where dislocations occur. Exercises should strengthen muscles while joints are positioned near their end ranges.

Closed-chain exercises provide joint stability through weight-bearing positions that compress joints and require muscular co-contractions. Examples include wall pushes, modified planks, and supported squats. These exercises are generally safer than open-chain movements that allow joints to move freely through space.

Muscle Activation Patterns

Hypermobile joints often develop compensatory movement patterns where some muscles become overactive while others become inhibited. Overactive muscles may feel tight despite actually being weak, while inhibited muscles fail to provide adequate joint support.

Core stabilization takes on special importance in hypermobility because the deep stabilizing muscles often fail to activate properly. These muscles—including the diaphragm, pelvic floor, and deep abdominals—work together to provide internal stability that supports all movement patterns.

Timing sequencing of muscle activation affects joint stability and movement efficiency. In healthy movement, stabilizing muscles activate before prime movers, but this sequence is often disrupted in hypermobility. Training should focus on activating stabilizers before adding movement or resistance.

Eccentric strengthening targets the lengthening phase of muscle contractions, which is particularly important for controlling hypermobile joints. Eccentric exercises teach muscles to control movement as joints move through their excessive ranges of motion.

Movement Quality Assessment

Compensation patterns develop when the body finds ways to move despite poor joint stability. These patterns may allow function in the short term but often lead to pain and injury over time. Common compensations include excessive spinal movement to make up for limited hip mobility or shoulder elevation during arm movements.

Neutral positioning becomes a learned skill for people with hypermobility because "normal" joint positions may feel uncomfortable or unstable. Learning to find and maintain neutral spine, hip, and shoulder positions forms the foundation for safe movement.

Movement efficiency improves when joints move within optimal ranges rather than excessive ranges. This often means learning to move less rather than more, using smaller ranges of motion that maintain joint stability.

Fatigue monitoring helps identify when movement quality deteriorates and injury risk increases. Hypermobile individuals often experience rapid onset of muscle fatigue that leads to loss of joint control. Exercise sessions should end before significant fatigue affects movement quality.

Heart Rate Monitoring for POTS

Traditional heart rate training zones don't apply to people with POTS, whose heart rates may spike unpredictably or remain elevated throughout activity. Understanding your individual heart rate patterns guides safe exercise intensity.

Individualized Heart Rate Zones

Resting heart rate establishment requires consistent measurement under similar conditions because POTS patients often have variable resting rates. Measure heart rate upon waking, before getting out of bed, for several days to establish your baseline.

Orthostatic heart rate changes should be measured regularly because they can vary based on hydration, medication timing, and overall health status. Stand for 10 minutes while monitoring heart rate to understand your typical postural responses.

Exercise heart rate targets focus on avoiding excessive increases rather than reaching specific training zones. Many POTS patients need to keep exercise heart rates within 20-30 beats per minute of their standing resting rate to avoid symptoms.

Recovery monitoring tracks how quickly heart rate returns to baseline after activity. Poor recovery—heart rate remaining elevated for more than 10-15 minutes after light activity—indicates that exercise intensity was too high or that overall condition is declining.

Technology Integration

Wearable devices provide real-time feedback that helps you stay within safe heart rate ranges during activity. Choose devices that can be set to alert you when heart rate exceeds predetermined thresholds. Some devices also track heart rate variability, which may provide additional insights into autonomic function.

Smartphone apps can log exercise sessions and track patterns over time. Look for apps that allow you to record subjective symptoms alongside objective heart rate data. This combination helps identify relationships between heart rate patterns and symptom experiences.

Bluetooth chest straps often provide more accurate heart rate monitoring than wrist-based devices, especially during exercise when arm movement can interfere with wrist sensors. The improved accuracy helps you make better decisions about exercise intensity.

Data analysis over time reveals patterns that aren't obvious from individual exercise sessions. Weekly and monthly reviews of heart rate data help identify improvements in exercise tolerance or warning signs of declining condition.

Symptom Recognition During Exercise

Early warning signs of POTS episodes during exercise include sudden heart rate spikes, lightheadedness, visual changes, nausea, or excessive fatigue. Learning to recognize these signs allows you to stop exercise before symptoms become severe.

Safe stopping procedures involve gradually reducing intensity rather than stopping abruptly, which can trigger rebound hypotension. Walk slowly or perform gentle movements while heart rate gradually returns to baseline.

Position modifications during exercise can prevent or minimize POTS symptoms. Recumbent or horizontal exercises avoid the gravitational challenges that trigger orthostatic intolerance. Semi-reclined positions provide compromise between upright exercise and symptom management.

Hydration timing affects exercise tolerance in POTS patients. Pre-exercise hydration with electrolyte solutions can improve performance, while dehydration significantly worsens symptoms. Monitor fluid losses during exercise and replace appropriately.

Progressive Loading Principles

Building exercise tolerance in trifecta patients requires gradual progressions that allow adaptation without triggering setbacks. The traditional approach of linear progression often doesn't work for people with chronic illness.

Gradual Intensity Increases

Starting intensities should be well below what you think you can tolerate because chronic illness often impairs accurate perception of exertion. Begin with activities that feel almost too easy—this conservative approach prevents setbacks that can derail progress.

Weekly progressions focus on small increases in duration before increasing intensity. Add 2-3 minutes to exercise sessions each week rather than increasing intensity or resistance. Duration tolerance often improves faster than intensity tolerance in chronic illness.

Plateau periods are normal and necessary parts of progression for people with chronic illness. Plan for periods where you maintain current activity levels without increases. These consolidation phases allow your body to adapt fully before adding new challenges.

Regression protocols help you respond appropriately when symptoms worsen or life stressors increase. Having predetermined plans for reducing exercise intensity prevents abandonment of all activity during difficult periods.

Load Tolerance Development

Resistance progression for hypermobile joints focuses on improving muscular endurance and control rather than maximum strength. High-repetition, low-resistance exercises build the sustained muscle activation needed for joint stability.

Time under tension becomes more important than total resistance for people with hypermobility. Slower movements that require sustained muscle contractions improve neuromuscular control and joint stability better than fast, high-weight movements.

Functional movement patterns should form the foundation of strength training rather than isolated muscle exercises. Movements that integrate multiple joints and muscle groups better translate to improved daily function.

Recovery monitoring between sessions helps determine appropriate training frequency. People with chronic illness often need longer recovery periods between exercise sessions. Schedule rest days proactively rather than exercising until exhaustion forces time off.

Adaptation Monitoring

Positive adaptations in chronic illness may be subtle and take longer to appear than in healthy populations. Track functional improvements like climbing stairs with less fatigue or standing for longer periods without symptoms, rather than focusing only on traditional fitness measures.

Warning signs of overtraining include worsening sleep, increased resting heart rate, elevated morning symptoms, or prolonged recovery from exercise sessions. These signs indicate need for immediate reduction in exercise intensity or frequency.

Plateau recognition helps distinguish between normal adaptation periods and signs of overreaching. Planned plateau periods are beneficial, while unexpected loss of progress may indicate excessive training stress.

Program modifications should be made based on overall trends rather than day-to-day fluctuations. Chronic illness creates normal variability in daily function, so programming decisions should consider patterns over weeks rather than individual sessions.

Activity Modification Strategies

Most recreational and sports activities can be modified to accommodate trifecta conditions with creativity and proper planning. The goal is maintaining participation in enjoyable activities while managing medical limitations.

Sports Adaptation Principles

Contact sports modifications focus on protecting hypermobile joints from sudden impacts or movements that could cause dislocations. Bracing, protective equipment, and rule modifications can allow participation in many sports with reduced injury risk.

Team sport accommodations might include position changes that reduce running requirements, modified rules that account for exercise limitations, or substitute players who can rotate in during symptom episodes.

Individual sport modifications often work better for people with unpredictable symptoms because pacing can be self-controlled. Golf, swimming, cycling, and tennis can often be modified to accommodate various limitations.

Competitive considerations require honest assessment of risk versus benefit. Some level of competition may be possible with appropriate modifications, while high-level competition might be incompatible with chronic illness management.

Equipment and Environmental Modifications

Assistive equipment can extend participation in many activities beyond what would be possible without support. Braces, taping, and supportive clothing can provide joint stability during activity.

Environmental controls help manage triggers that might interfere with exercise tolerance. Air conditioning, air filtration, and climate control can reduce MCAS triggers during indoor activities.

Timing modifications work around predictable symptom patterns and medication effects. Schedule activities during your best times of day and coordinate with medication timing for optimal performance.

Location alternatives provide backup options when primary exercise venues aren't suitable. Home exercise equipment, multiple gym memberships, or outdoor alternatives ensure you can maintain activity despite changing circumstances.

The Recumbent Revolution

Horizontal and semi-reclined exercise positions can provide significant cardiovascular and strength benefits while minimizing orthostatic stress from POTS. These positions work with your physiology rather than against it.

Recumbent Cardiovascular Training

Recumbent bikes eliminate the postural challenges that make upright cycling difficult for POTS patients. The horizontal position supports venous return and reduces heart rate elevation, allowing for longer, more comfortable exercise sessions.

Rowing machines provide full-body cardiovascular exercise in a seated position that supports the torso. The pulling motion strengthens postural muscles while providing cardiovascular benefits without orthostatic stress.

Swimming offers ideal cardiovascular exercise for trifecta patients because the horizontal position and hydrostatic pressure support circulation. Water temperature should be kept moderate to avoid triggering MCAS reactions or excessive heart rate responses.

Supine exercises include various movements that can be performed lying down while still providing cardiovascular benefits. Examples include leg cycling movements, arm exercises with resistance bands, and modified calisthenics.

Strength Training Adaptations

Floor exercises provide stable positions for strength training that don't challenge postural control systems. Many traditional exercises can be modified for floor positions without losing effectiveness.

Supported positions using walls, chairs, or exercise equipment provide stability for standing exercises when floor positions aren't practical. Wall pushes, chair-supported squats, and counter stretches work around stability limitations.

Resistance band training offers variable resistance that can be adjusted for different strength levels and joint limitations. Bands can be anchored at various heights to accommodate different positions and movement patterns.

Machine-based training provides external stability that supports proper form and reduces injury risk. Machines with back support are particularly beneficial for people with postural control difficulties.

Pool Therapy Protocols

Water-based exercise offers unique advantages for trifecta patients through hydrostatic pressure support, buoyancy assistance, and temperature regulation. The aquatic environment can make exercise possible when land-based activities are too challenging.

Aquatic Exercise Benefits

Hydrostatic pressure provides external compression that supports circulation and reduces heart rate response to exercise. This pressure effect can significantly improve exercise tolerance in POTS patients.

Buoyancy reduces joint loading while maintaining resistance for muscle strengthening. Water supports body weight, reducing stress on hypermobile joints while providing resistance for movement in all directions.

Temperature regulation through cool water can prevent overheating that triggers POTS and MCAS symptoms. Water temperature between 83-88°F typically provides optimal comfort for therapeutic exercise.

Graduated depth training allows progressive increase in gravitational challenge as tolerance improves. Starting in deeper water with more buoyancy support and gradually moving to shallower water provides natural progression.

Specific Aquatic Exercises

Water walking provides cardiovascular exercise with reduced impact and postural demands. Walking forward, backward, and sideways in chest-deep water challenges different muscle groups while maintaining support.

Resistance movements use water's natural resistance to strengthen muscles without requiring additional equipment. Pushing and pulling movements against water resistance provide strengthening in all planes of motion.

Balance training in water challenges proprioception while providing a safe environment for practicing stability skills. The support of water allows for more aggressive balance training than would be safe on land.

Flexibility work in warm water can help manage EDS-related muscle tension while avoiding overstretching hypermobile joints. Gentle movements in warm water promote relaxation without excessive joint mobility.

Pool Safety Considerations

Supervision recommendations become particularly important for people with unpredictable symptoms that could affect safety in water. Exercise with partners or in supervised environments when possible.

Entry and exit strategies should be planned to accommodate mobility limitations and prevent falls. Use pool lifts, gradual entry via steps, or partner assistance as needed.

Water quality considerations include chlorine sensitivity that might trigger MCAS reactions. Some patients tolerate salt water or outdoor pools better than heavily chlorinated indoor facilities.

Emergency procedures should be established for managing symptoms that occur during aquatic exercise. Know how to quickly exit the pool and have emergency contacts readily available.

Yoga and Stretching Adaptations

Traditional yoga and stretching can be problematic for hypermobile individuals, but modified approaches can provide benefits for flexibility, strength, and stress management without increasing joint instability.

Modified Yoga Principles

Strength-based yoga focuses on building muscular support around joints rather than increasing flexibility. Hold poses for shorter durations with emphasis on muscle activation rather than deepening stretches.

Prop usage provides external support that prevents joints from moving into excessive ranges of motion. Blocks, straps, and bolsters can modify poses to work within safe joint ranges.

Alignment emphasis teaches proper joint positioning and muscle activation patterns. Focus on neutral spine positions and balanced muscle engagement rather than achieving extreme pose variations.

Breath integration helps manage autonomic symptoms while providing stress relief benefits. Coordinate breathing patterns with movement to support nervous system regulation.

Safe Stretching Guidelines

Range limitations involve stopping stretches before reaching end-range joint positions. The goal is maintaining functional flexibility rather than maximum range of motion.

Muscle focus targets areas that tend to become tight due to compensatory movement patterns. Hip flexors, chest muscles, and neck muscles often need attention in people with postural adaptations.

Temperature considerations include warming muscles before stretching and using heat therapy when appropriate. Cold muscles and joints are more injury-prone in people with hypermobility.

Duration guidelines suggest shorter holds (15-30 seconds) rather than prolonged stretching that might increase joint laxity. Multiple shorter stretches may be more beneficial than single long holds.

Stress Management Integration

Meditation components of yoga practice provide stress management benefits without physical risks. Breathing exercises, guided imagery, and mindfulness practices support overall well-being.

Relaxation techniques help manage the chronic stress associated with living with chronic illness. Progressive muscle relaxation and body scan meditations can reduce muscle tension and improve sleep quality.

Mind-body connection development helps improve awareness of physical symptoms and stress responses. This awareness supports better self-management of chronic illness symptoms.

Community aspects of group yoga classes provide social support, though modifications may be needed to practice safely in group settings.

Working with Fitness Professionals

Finding trainers and therapists who understand chronic illness and hypermobility requires research and clear communication about your needs and limitations.

Trainer Selection Criteria

Chronic illness experience should be prioritized when selecting fitness professionals. Look for trainers who have worked with clients with chronic conditions and understand the need for modifications and variable progression.

Hypermobility knowledge helps trainers design appropriate exercise programs that focus on stability rather than mobility. Trainers with experience in corrective exercise or post-rehabilitation training often have relevant skills.

Communication skills are essential because you'll need to advocate for your needs and provide feedback about how exercises affect your symptoms. Look for professionals who listen to your concerns and adjust programs based on your responses.

Flexibility in programming allows for modifications based on daily symptom fluctuations and changing needs over time. Avoid trainers who insist on rigid programming that doesn't accommodate chronic illness variability.

Effective Communication Strategies

Medical information sharing helps fitness professionals understand your conditions and limitations. Provide written summaries of your diagnoses, medications, and any restrictions from your medical team.

Symptom reporting during sessions helps trainers understand your real-time responses to exercise. Be specific about what you're experiencing and how it differs from normal exercise sensations.

Boundary setting establishes clear limits about what you will and won't attempt during exercise sessions. Don't let trainers pressure you into activities that trigger symptoms or feel unsafe.

Progress communication includes both positive improvements and concerning symptoms that develop. Regular check-ins help trainers adjust programs based on your changing needs and responses.

Program Development Collaboration

Goal setting should focus on functional improvements and symptom management rather than traditional fitness metrics. Work with trainers to establish realistic, health-focused objectives.

Exercise selection prioritizes movements that support daily function and address specific impairments related to your conditions. Functional exercises often provide more benefit than traditional gym exercises.

Progression planning accounts for the variable nature of chronic illness and plans for both advancement and regression periods. Flexible programming prevents abandonment of exercise during symptom flares.

Monitoring systems track both objective measures (heart rate, exercise duration) and subjective experiences (energy levels, symptom responses) to guide program modifications.

Janet's physical therapy session, described at the beginning of this section, marked the start of her transformation from someone who feared movement to someone who used exercise as medicine. She learned to work within her body's limitations rather than against them, building strength and stability that improved her daily function while reducing pain and fatigue.

The journey from exercise frustration to exercise success requires patience, creativity, and willingness to abandon conventional fitness wisdom in favor of approaches that work for your unique physiology. The goal isn't to become an athlete—it's to use movement strategically to improve your symptoms, function, and quality of life.

Movement as Healing

Exercise for trifecta patients represents a fundamental shift from performance-oriented fitness to health-oriented movement. Success is measured not by how fast or how much you can do, but by how movement improves your daily life and long-term health outcomes.

The exercise habits you develop now will serve you throughout your life with chronic illness. Learning to listen to your body, modify activities appropriately, and maintain consistent movement despite symptoms creates a foundation for lifelong health and function.

Moving forward, the movement patterns and exercise tolerance you've developed support the sleep optimization strategies covered in the next section. Regular, appropriate exercise improves sleep quality while avoiding the overexertion that can interfere with restorative rest.

Fundamental Movement Principles for Trifecta Patients

- Exercise physiology for hypermobility focuses on building stability and control rather than increasing flexibility or range of motion

- Heart rate monitoring for POTS requires individualized zones that avoid orthostatic triggers while providing cardiovascular benefits

- Progressive loading must account for the variable nature of chronic illness with planned plateau and regression periods

- Activity modifications allow participation in enjoyable pursuits while managing medical limitations and injury risks

- Recumbent exercise positions provide cardiovascular and strength benefits while minimizing orthostatic stress

- Pool therapy offers unique advantages through hydrostatic pressure, buoyancy support, and temperature regulation

- Yoga and stretching adaptations emphasize strength and stability rather than increased flexibility for hypermobile joints

- Professional guidance requires finding trainers who understand chronic illness and can adapt programs to individual needs and limitations

Chapter 7: Sleep Architecture and Energy Economics

The sleep study technician frowned at the data streaming across her monitors as David lay connected to dozens of electrodes in the darkened laboratory. His heart rate, which should have decreased during sleep, instead showed a concerning pattern of elevation throughout the night. His breathing remained shallow and irregular, failing to achieve the deep, restorative patterns typical of healthy sleep. Most troubling, his autonomic nervous system showed signs of persistent activation—as if his body remained on high alert even during supposedly restful periods.

David's sleep study revealed what many trifecta patients experience but few understand: sleep that looks normal from the outside but fails to provide genuine restoration. His eight hours in bed included frequent micro-awakenings he didn't remember, periods of autonomic dysfunction that prevented deep sleep, and pain-related sleep fragmentation that left him exhausted despite adequate time for rest.

This sleep architecture disruption creates a cascade of problems that worsen all trifecta symptoms. Poor sleep increases inflammation, reduces pain tolerance, disrupts blood sugar regulation, and impairs immune function. It worsens POTS symptoms by affecting blood volume regulation and autonomic function. It triggers MCAS reactions by increasing stress hormones and reducing the body's ability to process allergens and toxins. It increases EDS-related pain by reducing the body's natural pain management systems.

Understanding sleep as a complex physiological process rather than simply "time in bed" transforms your approach to rest and recovery. Quality matters more than quantity, though both are important. The goal isn't just getting more sleep—it's optimizing sleep architecture to maximize the restorative processes that occur during different sleep stages.

Sleep Disorders in the Trifecta

Each trifecta condition affects sleep through different mechanisms, and these effects often compound each other to create complex sleep disruption patterns that require specialized management approaches.

POTS-Related Sleep Disruption

Autonomic dysfunction creates multiple barriers to quality sleep in POTS patients. The sympathetic nervous system, which should quiet during sleep to allow restoration, often remains hyperactive throughout the night. This persistent activation prevents the deep sleep stages necessary for physical recovery and cognitive restoration.

Heart rate fluctuations during sleep can cause frequent awakenings, even when patients don't consciously remember waking up. Sleep studies often reveal dozens of micro-awakenings throughout the night as the cardiovascular system struggles to maintain stable function in the supine position.

Blood pressure regulation becomes problematic during sleep transitions. Moving from lying down to sitting up for bathroom trips can trigger significant blood pressure drops that cause dizziness, nausea, or fainting. These episodes create anxiety about sleep that further disrupts rest patterns.

Temperature regulation fails to follow normal circadian patterns in many POTS patients. Core body temperature should drop during sleep preparation, but autonomic dysfunction can prevent this natural cooling process. Some patients experience night sweats while others feel persistently cold, both of which interfere with sleep quality.

Breathing pattern irregularities occur when autonomic dysfunction affects respiratory control during sleep. Shallow breathing, periodic breathing, or brief pauses in breathing can prevent achievement of deep sleep stages even when patients aren't aware of breathing difficulties.

MCAS Sleep Interference

Histamine release follows circadian patterns that can worsen at night, creating symptoms that interfere with sleep initiation and maintenance. Many patients experience increased itching, flushing, or respiratory symptoms during evening hours when histamine levels naturally peak.

Food reactions from dinner can trigger nighttime MCAS symptoms that prevent sleep or cause frequent awakenings. Delayed food reactions may not appear until 4-6 hours after eating, coinciding with bedtime and creating a pattern of nighttime symptoms that seems unrelated to food intake.

Environmental triggers in the bedroom often go unrecognized but can significantly affect sleep quality. Dust mites in bedding, off-gassing from synthetic materials, or cleaning product residues can trigger low-level MCAS reactions that prevent deep sleep without causing obvious symptoms.

Hormonal fluctuations affect mast cell stability throughout the menstrual cycle, with many women reporting worse sleep during specific cycle phases. Estrogen and progesterone changes can increase mast cell sensitivity and trigger reactions to previously tolerated exposures.

Medication timing affects sleep when antihistamines or other MCAS treatments are taken at inappropriate times. Some antihistamines can be sedating when taken at bedtime, while others may be stimulating and should be taken earlier in the day.

EDS Pain and Sleep Fragmentation

Joint pain intensifies during prolonged static positions like lying in bed, creating a cycle where rest increases pain that then prevents further rest. Finding comfortable sleeping positions becomes increasingly difficult as the night progresses and joints stiffen.

Subluxations and dislocations can occur during sleep when muscles relax and fail to provide adequate joint support. These injuries create sudden pain that causes awakening and anxiety about returning to sleep.

Soft tissue pain from muscle tension and fascial restrictions often worsens at night when the body attempts to relax. Paradoxically, the relaxation process can increase awareness of chronic pain that was masked by daytime activities.

Cervical instability creates particular problems for sleep quality when neck support is inadequate. Poor cervical alignment during sleep can affect breathing, circulation, and nervous system function, creating symptoms that prevent restorative rest.

Chronic pain medications may provide relief but can also disrupt normal sleep architecture. Opioids in particular can reduce deep sleep and REM sleep, leading to non-restorative rest despite reduced pain levels.

Sleep Hygiene Plus - Advanced Strategies

Basic sleep hygiene recommendations provide starting points, but trifecta patients often need more sophisticated approaches that address the complex interactions between their conditions and sleep physiology.

Advanced Sleep Environment Optimization

Temperature control requires more precision than general recommendations for cool bedrooms. POTS patients may need gradual temperature reduction to avoid triggering autonomic responses, while MCAS patients may react to temperature extremes or rapid changes.

Air quality management becomes crucial when respiratory sensitivity affects sleep. HEPA air filtifiers, hypoallergenic bedding, and regular cleaning schedules can reduce environmental triggers that prevent quality rest.

Light exposure management involves more than just darkening the bedroom. Circadian rhythm disruption is common in chronic illness, requiring strategic light exposure timing to reset natural sleep-wake cycles.

Sound environment considerations include both obvious noise sources and subtle sounds that may trigger stress responses. White noise machines can mask household sounds while providing consistent auditory environments that support sleep maintenance.

Bedding selection affects both comfort and potential trigger exposure. Natural fiber bedding may reduce chemical exposures, while specific pillow and mattress types can provide better joint support for EDS patients.

Medication and Supplement Timing

Sleep medication optimization requires understanding how different drugs affect sleep architecture and interact with trifecta conditions. Some medications that induce sleep actually worsen sleep quality by preventing deep sleep stages.

Natural sleep aid timing becomes important when using supplements like melatonin, magnesium, or valerian. These supplements work best when taken at specific times relative to desired sleep onset and in appropriate dosages for individual needs.

POTS medication scheduling around bedtime can improve sleep quality when vasodilators or heart rate medications are timed to provide optimal coverage during sleep hours.

MCAS medication timing may require evening doses of antihistamines or mast cell stabilizers to prevent nighttime symptom flares that disrupt sleep.

Pain medication planning for EDS patients involves balancing pain relief with medication effects on sleep architecture. Some pain medications improve sleep by reducing discomfort, while others may impair sleep quality despite pain relief.

Pre-Sleep Routine Modifications

Gradual wind-down protocols help transition the nervous system from daytime activation to sleep preparation. This process may take longer for people with autonomic dysfunction and should begin 2-3 hours before desired sleep time.

Position transitions require planning for POTS patients who may experience symptoms when changing from upright to lying positions. Gradual transitions with intermediate reclining positions can minimize orthostatic symptoms.

Symptom management before bed includes addressing pain, respiratory symptoms, or anxiety that might interfere with sleep onset. Having management strategies in place prevents middle-of-the-night symptom episodes from derailing sleep.

Bathroom planning reduces the need for nighttime trips that can trigger POTS symptoms. Limiting fluids before bed and using the bathroom immediately before lying down can minimize sleep disruptions.

Environmental trigger reduction includes removing potential MCAS triggers from the bedroom and ensuring that evening meals don't contain reactive foods that might cause nighttime symptoms.

Energy Budgeting and Spoon Theory Application

Energy management for trifecta patients requires understanding that energy is a finite resource that must be budgeted carefully to accomplish necessary activities while preserving enough reserves for recovery and unexpected demands.

Understanding Energy Economics

Baseline energy assessment involves determining your daily energy capacity during stable periods. This baseline helps you understand how much energy you have available for activities and how much must be reserved for essential functions.

Energy expenditure tracking reveals which activities consume the most energy and helps identify areas where modifications might preserve energy for higher-priority tasks. Physical, cognitive, and emotional activities all draw from the same energy pool.

Recovery time calculation helps you understand how long it takes to replenish energy after different types of activities. This information guides scheduling and helps prevent the boom-bust cycles common in chronic illness.

Variable energy planning accounts for the fluctuating nature of energy levels in chronic illness. Good days and bad days require different approaches to activity planning and energy allocation.

Energy debt recognition helps you identify when you've exceeded your energy capacity and need focused recovery time. Energy debt creates symptoms that can take days or weeks to resolve if not addressed appropriately.

Practical Energy Management

Activity prioritization involves ranking daily tasks by importance and energy requirements. Essential activities like medication management and basic self-care take priority, while optional activities are scheduled based on available energy.

Task batching groups similar activities together to minimize energy spent on transitions and setup. Preparing all meals for the day at once or grouping errands into single trips can conserve energy.

Energy-saving modifications for routine activities can significantly reduce daily energy expenditure. Online shopping, meal delivery services, and household help can preserve energy for activities that can't be outsourced.

Rest scheduling involves planned breaks throughout the day rather than waiting until exhaustion forces rest. Strategic rest periods can prevent energy depletion and maintain higher function throughout the day.

Delegation strategies help distribute energy-consuming tasks among family members, friends, or hired help. Learning to accept help becomes a crucial skill for successful energy management.

Boom-Bust Cycle Prevention

Good day management prevents overexertion during periods of higher energy that lead to subsequent crashes. Planning moderate activity levels during good days helps maintain more consistent function over time.

Warning sign recognition helps identify early signs of energy depletion before severe symptoms develop. Fatigue, brain fog, increased pain, or mood changes may signal need for immediate rest.

Recovery protocols provide structured approaches to regaining energy after periods of overexertion. These protocols include specific rest activities, nutrition strategies, and medical interventions that support recovery.

Long-term pacing involves planning energy expenditure over weeks and months rather than just daily periods. Major events or activities may require energy conservation before and recovery time afterward.

Rest Versus Sleep - Understanding Recovery Types

Different types of rest provide different recovery benefits, and understanding these distinctions helps optimize recovery strategies for varying needs and energy levels.

Active Rest Strategies

Gentle movement during rest periods can improve circulation and prevent stiffness without consuming significant energy. Simple stretching, walking, or light yoga may be more restorative than complete inactivity.

Cognitive rest involves activities that provide mental relaxation without requiring concentration or decision-making. Listening to music, light reading, or watching familiar television shows can provide cognitive rest while remaining awake.

Social rest includes time spent with supportive people who understand your limitations and don't require energy expenditure for social performance. Quality time with understanding friends or family can be restorative rather than draining.

Creative rest engages different parts of the brain than daily responsibilities and can provide restoration through enjoyable activities. Art, music, writing, or crafts can be restful when approached without pressure or deadlines.

Passive Rest Techniques

Meditation and mindfulness practices provide mental rest while supporting nervous system regulation. Even short meditation sessions can provide significant restoration for people with chronic illness.

Progressive muscle relaxation helps reduce physical tension while providing mental rest. This technique can be particularly helpful for EDS patients who experience chronic muscle tension.

Breathing exercises support autonomic nervous system regulation and can provide both physical and mental restoration. Specific breathing patterns can activate the parasympathetic nervous system and promote recovery.

Visualization techniques provide mental escape and stress relief that can be restorative even when physical rest isn't possible. Guided imagery sessions can provide recovery benefits during busy periods.

Environmental Rest

Sensory reduction involves minimizing stimulation from light, sound, temperature, and other environmental factors that require energy to process. Creating quiet, comfortable environments supports deeper rest.

Technology breaks reduce the cognitive load and stimulation from electronic devices that can interfere with rest and recovery. Regular periods without screens can improve both rest quality and sleep preparation.

Nature exposure provides restoration through connection with natural environments that support nervous system regulation. Even viewing nature scenes through windows can provide restorative benefits.

Routine simplification reduces decision-making demands and cognitive load during rest periods. Having established routines for rest activities reduces energy expenditure on planning and decision-making.

Sleep Environment Optimization

Creating optimal sleep environments for trifecta patients requires attention to multiple environmental factors that can affect sleep quality and symptom management.

Temperature and Climate Control

Optimal temperature ranges for trifecta patients may be narrower than general recommendations due to autonomic dysfunction and increased environmental sensitivity. Most patients benefit from temperatures between 65-68°F, but individual preferences may vary.

Humidity control helps prevent respiratory symptoms and skin irritation that can interfere with sleep. Humidity levels between 30-50% typically provide optimal comfort for most people with chronic illness.

Air circulation prevents stagnant air that can worsen respiratory symptoms or trigger reactions to environmental allergens. Ceiling fans or air circulation systems can improve air quality without creating drafts.

Heating and cooling system maintenance prevents mold growth and reduces airborne irritants that might trigger MCAS reactions during sleep. Regular filter changes and system cleaning are particularly important for sensitive individuals.

Lighting and Circadian Support

Blackout solutions block external light sources that can interfere with melatonin production and circadian rhythm regulation. Room-darkening shades, blackout curtains, or eye masks can improve sleep quality.

Blue light reduction in the evening supports natural melatonin production. Blue light blocking glasses or device filters can help maintain circadian rhythms when evening screen use is necessary.

Morning light exposure helps reset circadian rhythms and improve daytime alertness. Natural sunlight or bright therapy lights used consistently in the morning can improve overall sleep-wake cycles.

Nighttime lighting for safety should provide minimal illumination for necessary movement without disrupting sleep. Red-tinted nightlights preserve night vision while providing safety lighting.

Noise Management

Sound masking using white noise, brown noise, or nature sounds can block disruptive noises while providing consistent auditory environments that support sleep maintenance.

Noise isolation through window treatments, door seals, or bedroom location selection can reduce external noise disturbances that might cause sleep fragmentation.

Household noise management involves coordinating family activities and schedules to minimize disruptions during sleep hours. Communication with family members about sleep needs is essential.

Technology noise includes electronic device sounds, HVAC system noise, and electrical interference that might be subtle but disruptive to sensitive individuals.

Medication Timing and Sleep Coordination

Coordinating medication schedules with sleep cycles can improve both drug effectiveness and sleep quality while minimizing side effects that interfere with rest.

POTS Medication Sleep Considerations

Beta-blockers may improve sleep by reducing heart rate variability but can also cause vivid dreams or nightmares in some patients. Timing these medications appropriately can maximize benefits while minimizing sleep disruption.

Fludrocortisone timing affects fluid retention and blood pressure regulation throughout the day. Taking this medication in the morning helps maintain blood volume during waking hours while minimizing nighttime fluid retention.

Vasodilators may cause nighttime hypotension if taken too close to bedtime. Spacing these medications appropriately prevents dangerous blood pressure drops during sleep.

Stimulant medications used for fatigue must be timed carefully to avoid interfering with sleep onset. These medications should typically be taken in the morning and early afternoon only.

MCAS Medication Sleep Effects

Antihistamine timing affects both symptom control and sleep quality. Sedating antihistamines can be helpful when taken at bedtime, while non-sedating varieties should be taken earlier in the day.

Mast cell stabilizers may need to be taken in divided doses to provide 24-hour coverage that includes nighttime symptom prevention.

Leukotriene inhibitors can be activating for some patients and may interfere with sleep if taken too close to bedtime.

Corticosteroid timing significantly affects sleep quality. These medications should be taken in the morning to minimize sleep disruption from their stimulating effects.

Pain Medication Sleep Balance

Opioid medications can provide pain relief that improves sleep comfort but may also disrupt sleep architecture by reducing deep sleep and REM sleep stages.

Non-opioid pain medications like gabapentin or pregabalin may actually improve sleep quality in addition to providing pain relief.

Topical pain medications can provide localized relief without systemic effects that might interfere with sleep.

Timing pain medications to provide peak coverage during typical pain exacerbation periods can improve sleep quality without overmedication.

Nap Strategy and Timing

Strategic napping can improve function and energy levels for trifecta patients, but poor nap timing or duration can interfere with nighttime sleep and worsen overall sleep quality.

Optimal Nap Timing

Early afternoon naps between 1-3 PM align with natural circadian rhythm dips and are less likely to interfere with nighttime sleep than later naps.

Duration limitations of 20-30 minutes prevent entry into deep sleep stages that can cause grogginess upon awakening and interfere with nighttime sleep drive.

Individual timing optimization requires tracking how different nap times affect your nighttime sleep quality and overall energy levels.

Activity-based napping involves timing naps before challenging activities that require higher energy levels, rather than napping only when exhausted.

Nap Environment Optimization

Position considerations for trifecta patients include supporting hypermobile joints during naps and using positions that don't trigger POTS symptoms upon awakening.

Environmental consistency between nap and nighttime sleep environments can improve nap quality and support overall sleep hygiene.

Wake-up strategies prevent the grogginess that can follow naps by using gentle alarm systems and light exposure to support alertness upon awakening.

Nap replacement activities provide alternatives to napping when sleep timing would interfere with nighttime rest. Quiet rest, meditation, or gentle activities can provide restoration without sleep.

Managing Nap Dependencies

Reducing nap dependence involves gradually improving nighttime sleep quality so that daytime naps become optional rather than necessary.

Nap scheduling prevents random napping that can disrupt circadian rhythms and interfere with consistent sleep-wake cycles.

Energy management alternatives to napping include rest breaks, stress reduction, and activity modification that provide restoration without sleep.

Medical evaluation for excessive nap needs may reveal underlying sleep disorders or medical issues that require specific treatment.

Sleep Study Considerations

Sleep studies can provide valuable information about sleep architecture and identify treatable sleep disorders, but preparation and interpretation require special considerations for trifecta patients.

Preparing for Sleep Studies

Medication management during sleep studies requires coordination with sleep specialists about which medications to continue or discontinue before testing.

Environmental preparation involves discussing accommodation needs for MCAS triggers, temperature sensitivity, or positioning requirements during overnight studies.

Expectation setting helps prepare for the artificial nature of sleep laboratory environments that may not reflect normal sleep patterns.

Home sleep studies may provide more accurate information for some patients whose symptoms are triggered by unfamiliar environments or medical settings.

Interpreting Results

Sleep architecture analysis reveals how much time is spent in different sleep stages and whether restorative deep sleep and REM sleep are occurring adequately.

Respiratory findings may reveal sleep apnea, upper airway resistance, or breathing pattern disorders that contribute to poor sleep quality.

Movement disorders during sleep, including periodic limb movements or restless leg syndrome, can significantly fragment sleep and contribute to fatigue.

Autonomic findings may show heart rate variability, blood pressure changes, or other signs of autonomic dysfunction during sleep.

Treatment Implementation

CPAP therapy for sleep apnea requires special considerations for patients with MCAS who may react to mask materials or cleaning products.

Medication adjustments based on sleep study findings should be coordinated with all members of your medical team to prevent interactions with existing treatments.

Lifestyle modifications recommended based on sleep studies should be integrated with existing chronic illness management strategies.

Follow-up studies may be needed to evaluate treatment effectiveness and monitor for changes in sleep patterns over time.

David's sleep study results, described at the beginning of this section, led to a comprehensive sleep optimization program that addressed his autonomic dysfunction, environmental triggers, and pain management needs. His sleep quality improved gradually over several months as he implemented multiple strategies simultaneously rather than focusing on single interventions.

The transformation from poor sleep to restorative rest requires patience and multifaceted approaches that address the complex interactions between trifecta conditions and sleep physiology. Sleep improvement often provides the foundation that supports progress in all other areas of chronic illness management.

Sleep as Restoration Foundation

Quality sleep provides the foundation that supports immune function, pain management, cognitive performance, and emotional regulation. For trifecta patients, optimizing sleep architecture often produces improvements that extend far beyond feeling more rested.

The sleep strategies you develop become lifelong skills that adapt to changing needs as your conditions evolve. Understanding sleep as an active process rather than passive downtime empowers you to take control of this crucial aspect of health management.

Moving forward, the energy management skills and sleep optimization you've achieved create the foundation for the more advanced treatment approaches and lifestyle integration strategies covered in upcoming sections. Quality sleep and effective energy management make everything else possible.

Core Sleep and Energy Management Concepts

- Sleep disorders in trifecta conditions involve complex interactions between autonomic dysfunction, immune activation, and chronic pain

- Advanced sleep hygiene strategies address the specific environmental and physiological challenges faced by chronic illness patients

- Energy budgeting using spoon theory principles prevents boom-bust cycles and maintains more consistent daily function

- Different types of rest provide various recovery benefits and should be used strategically based on individual needs

- Sleep environment optimization requires attention to temperature, lighting, air quality, and noise factors that affect sensitive individuals

- Medication timing coordination with sleep cycles improves both treatment effectiveness and sleep quality

- Strategic napping can enhance function when timed and structured appropriately to avoid nighttime sleep interference

- Sleep studies provide valuable diagnostic information but require special preparation and interpretation for trifecta patients

Chapter 8: Pharmaceutical Orchestra

Coordinating Complex Medication Regimens

The pharmacy counter looked like a small battlefield as Rachel spread out seventeen different prescription bottles, three over-the-counter supplements, and a handwritten medication schedule that resembled a complex musical score. Her pharmacist, Dr. Martinez, studied the array with the focused attention of a conductor preparing for a symphony performance. "This metoprolol for your POTS," he said, pointing to one bottle, "peaks about two hours after you take it, right when your cromolyn sodium is starting to work for MCAS. But if you take them together, the metoprolol might reduce the absorption of the cromolyn."

Rachel's medication regimen represented what many trifecta patients face—a complex orchestra of drugs that must work together harmoniously while avoiding discordant interactions. Each condition requires specific medications, but these drugs don't exist in isolation. They interact with each other, compete for absorption pathways, affect the same metabolic systems, and create timing challenges that would challenge even experienced physicians.

The stakes for getting this right are high. Poorly coordinated medication regimens can worsen symptoms, create dangerous interactions, or render treatments ineffective. A beta-blocker taken at the wrong time might prevent a mast cell stabilizer from working properly. An antihistamine might mask early warning signs of a serious reaction. Pain medications might worsen orthostatic intolerance.

Success requires thinking like a conductor who must coordinate multiple instrument sections to create beautiful music rather than cacophonous noise. You need to understand what each medication does, when it works best, how it interacts with others, and how to time everything for maximum therapeutic benefit with minimum side effects.

Medication Categories for Trifecta Management

Understanding drug classes helps you see the bigger picture of how different medications work together rather than viewing each prescription as an isolated treatment. Each category affects your body systems differently and requires specific timing and monitoring considerations.

POTS Medication Classes

Beta-blockers form the foundation of POTS treatment for many patients by reducing heart rate response to position changes and activity. Metoprolol, propranolol, and atenolol work by blocking beta-adrenergic receptors, but they differ in their selectivity, duration of action, and side effect profiles (13).

These medications typically reach peak effectiveness 1-3 hours after oral administration and last 6-12 hours depending on the specific drug and formulation. Extended-release versions provide more consistent blood levels but may be less flexible for dose adjustments.

Mineralocorticoids like fludrocortisone help retain sodium and expand blood volume, addressing one of the underlying mechanisms of POTS. This medication works slowly, taking days to weeks for full effect, and requires careful monitoring of blood pressure and electrolyte levels (14).

Fludrocortisone is typically taken once daily in the morning because it can cause fluid retention that interferes with sleep if taken later in the day. The dose usually starts low and increases gradually based on symptom response and blood pressure tolerance.

Alpha-agonists such as midodrine provide direct vasoconstriction that helps maintain blood pressure during position changes. These medications have a rapid onset but short duration, requiring multiple daily doses spaced 3-4 hours apart (15).

The timing of midodrine doses is critical because the medication can cause supine hypertension if taken too close to bedtime. Most patients take their last dose at least 4 hours before lying down for the night.

MCAS Medication Arsenal

H1 antihistamines like cetirizine, loratadine, and fexofenadine block histamine receptors that cause allergic symptoms. These medications vary in their sedating effects, duration of action, and ability to cross the blood-brain barrier (16).

Non-sedating antihistamines work best when taken consistently rather than as needed because they prevent mast cell mediator effects rather than just treating symptoms after they occur. Timing with meals can affect absorption for some of these medications.

H2 antihistamines such as famotidine and ranitidine block different histamine receptors, particularly in the digestive system. These medications complement H1 antihistamines and may provide additional symptom relief when used together (17).

H2 blockers are often taken twice daily and may be more effective when taken before meals to prevent food-related reactions. Some patients find that H2 blockers help with sleep when taken at bedtime.

Mast cell stabilizers like cromolyn sodium work differently than antihistamines by preventing mast cells from releasing their inflammatory mediators. These medications must be taken consistently to build up tissue levels and are most effective when taken before meals (18).

Cromolyn sodium has poor oral bioavailability and works primarily in the digestive tract where it's taken. The timing relative to meals is crucial for effectiveness, and patients often need to experiment with timing to find what works best.

Leukotriene inhibitors such as montelukast block inflammatory pathways that complement histamine effects. These medications are typically taken once daily and may be particularly helpful for respiratory and skin symptoms (19).

EDS Pain Management Categories

Neuropathic pain medications like gabapentin and pregabalin target nerve-related pain that's common in EDS patients. These medications require gradual dose increases and consistent timing to maintain steady blood levels (20).

These drugs can cause sedation and cognitive effects, so timing relative to daily activities becomes important. Many patients find that taking larger doses at bedtime helps with both pain and sleep.

NSAIDs (non-steroidal anti-inflammatory drugs) provide anti-inflammatory effects that can help with joint pain and inflammation. However, EDS patients may be more prone to gastrointestinal side effects and should use these medications carefully (21).

The timing of NSAIDs relative to meals and other medications affects both effectiveness and side effect risk. Taking them with food reduces stomach irritation but may slightly delay absorption.

Muscle relaxants like cyclobenzaprine and tizanidine help with muscle spasms and tension that develop as compensation for joint instability. These medications often cause sedation and are typically taken at bedtime (22).

Topical pain medications provide localized relief without systemic effects that might interact with other medications. These can be particularly useful for targeting specific painful joints or areas.

Interaction Awareness and Management

Drug interactions in trifecta patients go beyond simple incompatibility warnings—they involve complex relationships between medications that affect absorption, metabolism, effectiveness, and side effects.

Absorption Interactions

Timing-dependent interactions occur when medications compete for absorption pathways or when one drug affects the absorption of another. Calcium supplements can reduce the absorption of certain antibiotics, while iron supplements may interfere with thyroid medication absorption (23).

Food effects vary significantly between medications and can either enhance or reduce absorption. Some medications must be taken on an empty stomach for optimal absorption, while others require food to prevent stomach irritation or improve bioavailability.

pH-dependent interactions become important when patients take acid-reducing medications for MCAS symptoms. Proton pump inhibitors and H2 blockers can affect the absorption of medications that require acidic conditions for dissolution.

Binding interactions occur when medications or supplements physically bind to each other in the digestive tract, preventing absorption. Calcium, iron, and magnesium supplements are particularly prone to these interactions.

Metabolic Interactions

Liver enzyme interactions affect how quickly medications are broken down and eliminated from the body. Some medications increase enzyme activity, making other drugs less effective, while others decrease enzyme activity, potentially causing toxic accumulation (24).

Common enzyme inducers include certain seizure medications and herbal supplements like St. John's wort. These can increase the metabolism of other medications, requiring dose adjustments to maintain effectiveness.

Enzyme inhibitors like certain antifungal medications and some antibiotics can slow the metabolism of other drugs, potentially causing side effects or toxic effects even at normal doses.

Genetic variations in liver enzymes affect how individuals metabolize certain medications. Pharmacogenetic testing can help identify patients who are poor or rapid metabolizers of specific drug classes.

Pharmacodynamic Interactions

Additive effects occur when multiple medications affect the same body systems in similar ways. Multiple sedating medications can cause excessive sleepiness, while several blood pressure medications might cause dangerous hypotension.

Antagonistic effects happen when medications work against each other's therapeutic effects. Beta-blockers might reduce the effectiveness of bronchodilators, while NSAIDs can interfere with blood pressure medications.

Receptor competition occurs when medications compete for the same receptor sites. This can reduce the effectiveness of both medications or create unpredictable responses.

Case Study: Complex Interaction Management

Maria, a 34-year-old with all three trifecta conditions, experienced worsening symptoms despite taking appropriate medications. Her regimen included metoprolol for POTS, cetirizine and famotidine for MCAS, and gabapentin for EDS-related pain.

Investigation revealed that she was taking all medications together with breakfast, including a calcium supplement for bone health. The calcium was reducing absorption of several medications, while the timing meant that peak drug levels didn't align with her symptom patterns.

Working with her pharmacist, Maria restructured her medication schedule. She took metoprolol and gabapentin with breakfast, moved her antihistamines to mid-morning on an empty stomach, took famotidine before lunch and dinner, and shifted calcium to bedtime when it wouldn't interfere with other medications.

This timing optimization, without changing any doses or medications, resulted in significant symptom improvement within two weeks. Her POTS symptoms became more predictable, MCAS reactions decreased in frequency and severity, and her pain levels became more manageable.

Timing and Spacing Optimization

Strategic medication timing can significantly improve therapeutic effectiveness while reducing side effects. This requires understanding each medication's onset, peak effect, duration, and how these factors relate to your symptom patterns.

Peak Effect Coordination

Onset timing varies dramatically between medications and affects when you'll notice therapeutic effects. Some medications like midodrine work within 30 minutes, while others like fludrocortisone may take weeks to show full effects.

Peak concentration timing determines when medications provide maximum benefit. Coordinating peak effects with times when you need maximum symptom control can improve quality of life and functional capacity.

Duration planning helps ensure continuous coverage for symptoms that require ongoing management while avoiding medication overlap that might cause side effects.

Half-life considerations affect how frequently medications need to be taken and how long they remain in your system.

Understanding half-lives helps plan dose timing and predict when medications will clear your system.

Circadian Rhythm Integration

Natural rhythm alignment involves timing medications to work with your body's natural daily cycles. Cortisol-like medications work best when taken in the morning to mimic natural hormone patterns.

Sleep consideration requires avoiding stimulating medications near bedtime while ensuring that pain medications provide adequate overnight coverage.

Activity coordination aligns medication peak effects with times when you need maximum symptom control for work, exercise, or social activities.

Symptom pattern matching involves timing medications based on when specific symptoms are typically worst. POTS symptoms often worsen in late afternoon, while pain may be worst upon waking.

Meal Timing Relationships

Food requirements vary by medication and affect both absorption and tolerability. Some medications must be taken with food to prevent stomach upset, while others require empty stomach conditions for optimal absorption.

Nutritional interactions can affect medication effectiveness. Vitamin K-rich foods can interfere with blood thinners, while calcium-rich foods may reduce absorption of certain antibiotics.

Digestive timing becomes important for MCAS patients who may have gastroparesis or delayed gastric emptying that affects medication absorption patterns.

MCAS trigger foods can affect medication absorption and effectiveness if reactions cause digestive symptoms around the time medications are taken.

Side Effect Management and Recognition

Distinguishing between medication side effects and disease symptoms requires careful observation and systematic tracking. This skill becomes essential for optimizing treatment while avoiding unnecessary medication changes.

Common Side Effect Patterns

Cardiovascular effects from multiple medications can compound to cause problematic blood pressure or heart rate changes. Beta-blockers lower heart rate and blood pressure, while some MCAS medications might have opposite effects.

Cognitive effects from multiple sources can impair function and quality of life. Antihistamines, pain medications, and some POTS treatments can all cause brain fog or drowsiness that may be difficult to distinguish from disease-related cognitive symptoms.

Gastrointestinal effects affect many trifecta medications and can worsen symptoms that are already problematic due to disease processes. NSAIDs can cause stomach irritation, while some MCAS treatments might affect appetite or digestion.

Sleep disturbances can result from medication timing, stimulating effects, or sedating effects that don't align with natural sleep patterns.

Timing-Related Side Effects

Peak-related side effects occur when medication levels are highest and may be manageable by adjusting dose timing or using extended-release formulations.

Withdrawal effects can occur when medications wear off before the next dose, particularly with short-acting medications or when doses are missed.

Cumulative effects develop over time as medications build up in your system or as your body adapts to treatment. These effects may not be apparent immediately after starting treatment.

Interaction-related side effects result from drug combinations and may not occur with individual medications alone.

Documentation and Tracking

Symptom timing relative to medication doses helps identify whether problems are medication-related or disease-related. Symptoms that consistently occur at specific times relative to doses suggest medication effects.

Dose-response relationships help distinguish between side effects and inadequate treatment. Increasing symptoms with higher doses suggest side effects, while persistent symptoms despite adequate doses may indicate need for different approaches.

Rechallenge testing involves temporarily stopping suspected medications to see if symptoms improve, then restarting to see if symptoms return. This should only be done under medical supervision.

Alternative explanations should be considered before attributing symptoms to medications. Disease progression, new triggers, stress, or other factors might explain symptom changes.

Pharmacy Relationships and Partnerships

Building strong relationships with knowledgeable pharmacists can significantly improve your medication management and safety. Pharmacists often have more time than physicians to discuss drug interactions and timing optimization.

Selecting the Right Pharmacy

Chronic illness experience matters when choosing a pharmacy because complex medication regimens require pharmacists who understand drug interactions and timing issues beyond basic safety checks.

Specialized services like medication synchronization, compliance packaging, and clinical consultation can significantly improve medication management for people with complex regimens.

Technology capabilities including electronic health record integration, medication reminder systems, and drug interaction screening can prevent problems before they occur.

Staff consistency allows you to build relationships with pharmacists who understand your specific medication needs and can provide personalized guidance.

Maximizing Pharmacy Services

Medication reviews involve comprehensive evaluations of your entire medication regimen to identify potential interactions, timing issues, or optimization opportunities.

Drug interaction screening goes beyond basic computer alerts to include consideration of timing, doses, and individual patient factors that affect interaction risk.

Dosing optimization may reveal opportunities to improve effectiveness or reduce side effects through timing changes, formulation switches, or dose adjustments.

Cost optimization includes identifying generic alternatives, therapeutic substitutions, or patient assistance programs that can reduce medication expenses.

Communication Strategies

Complete medication lists should include all prescription medications, over-the-counter drugs, supplements, and herbal products. Even seemingly minor supplements can interact with prescription medications.

Symptom reporting helps pharmacists understand how medications are affecting you and identify potential problems or optimization opportunities.

Goal clarification ensures that your pharmacist understands your treatment priorities and can make recommendations that align with your objectives.

Follow-up scheduling provides opportunities to assess medication effectiveness and make adjustments based on your response to treatment.

Generic Versus Brand Considerations

The decision between generic and brand-name medications becomes more complex for trifecta patients because small differences in formulation can affect symptom management in ways that aren't problematic for healthy individuals.

Bioequivalence Understanding

FDA standards require generic medications to be bioequivalent to brand-name versions, meaning they must deliver the same amount of active ingredient to the bloodstream within acceptable ranges—typically 80-125% of the brand-name product (25).

For most medications and most patients, this variation is clinically insignificant. However, trifecta patients may be more sensitive to small changes in drug levels due to their underlying physiological instability.

Narrow therapeutic index medications require more precise dosing because small changes in blood levels can affect effectiveness or cause side effects. Some POTS and seizure medications fall into this category.

Individual sensitivity varies, and some patients may notice differences between generic and brand formulations while others experience no difference at all.

Formulation Differences

Inactive ingredients in generic medications may differ from brand-name versions and can affect absorption, tolerability, or trigger MCAS reactions in sensitive patients.

Release characteristics can vary between immediate-release, extended-release, and different generic formulations, potentially affecting timing of therapeutic effects.

Excipient sensitivity affects some MCAS patients who react to specific inactive ingredients like dyes, preservatives, or binding agents used in medication manufacturing.

Coating materials and capsule compositions can trigger reactions in highly sensitive individuals, making brand-name medications necessary despite higher costs.

Cost-Benefit Analysis

Insurance coverage often favors generic medications, but some plans allow brand-name coverage with prior authorization when medical necessity is documented.

Price differences can be substantial, with brand-name medications sometimes costing 10-20 times more than generic equivalents.

Patient assistance programs from pharmaceutical manufacturers may make brand-name medications affordable for patients who meet income requirements.

Long-term costs should consider not just medication prices but also the cost of managing symptoms if generic formulations are less effective.

Practical Decision Framework

Trial periods with generic medications can help determine if they're as effective as brand-name versions without committing to long-term use.

Objective monitoring using symptom tracking, heart rate data, or other measurable parameters can help assess whether formulation changes affect therapeutic outcomes.

Medical team consultation helps ensure that decisions about generic versus brand medications are made with input from physicians who understand your specific medical needs.

Pharmacy communication about generic manufacturers can help maintain consistency by requesting specific generic brands that work well for you.

Travel Medication Planning

Managing trifecta medications while traveling requires advance planning to ensure medication access, TSA compliance, and maintenance of therapeutic regimens despite schedule disruptions.

TSA and Security Considerations

Prescription medications in original containers with pharmacy labels are allowed in both carry-on and checked luggage without quantity restrictions. However, carrying medications in original containers prevents confusion and potential delays.

Liquid medications over 3.4 ounces require separate screening but are allowed in carry-on luggage when declared at security checkpoints. This includes liquid supplements and compounded medications.

Medical documentation letters from physicians explaining medication needs can help with security screening and customs inspections, particularly for controlled substances or large quantities of medications.

Controlled substance regulations vary by destination country and may require special permits or documentation for international travel.

Supply Management

Extra medication supplies should account for travel delays, lost luggage, and difficulty accessing medications at your destination. Pack at least a week's extra supply of all essential medications.

Split supplies between carry-on and checked luggage to ensure access if one bag is lost. Never pack all medications in checked luggage only.

Prescription copies provide documentation for emergency refills and help international pharmacies understand your medication needs.

Time zone adjustments may require gradual schedule changes for medications that must be taken at specific intervals to maintain steady blood levels.

International Travel Considerations

Medication legality varies by country, and some medications available in the United States may be controlled or prohibited in other countries.

Generic name documentation helps international pharmacies identify equivalent medications if your specific formulations aren't available abroad.

Temperature stability becomes important for medications that require refrigeration or are sensitive to heat and humidity.

Emergency contact information for your medical team and pharmacy helps facilitate medication access if problems arise during travel.

Cost Management and Insurance Navigation

Trifecta patients often face significant medication costs due to the number of prescriptions required and the need for specific formulations that may not be preferred by insurance plans.

Insurance Optimization Strategies

Formulary understanding helps you and your medical team choose medications that are covered by your insurance plan while still providing appropriate treatment.

Prior authorization processes can be time-consuming but may provide coverage for non-preferred medications when medical necessity is documented.

Appeal procedures allow you to challenge insurance denials when covered medications are medically necessary for your conditions.

Step therapy requirements may require trying preferred medications before insurance will cover more expensive alternatives.

Patient Assistance Programs

Manufacturer programs provide free or reduced-cost medications for patients who meet income and insurance requirements. Most major pharmaceutical companies offer these programs.

Foundation grants from patient advocacy organizations may help cover medication costs for specific conditions or patient populations.

Pharmacy discount programs can reduce costs for patients without insurance or for medications not covered by insurance plans.

Government programs like Medicare Extra Help or state pharmaceutical assistance programs may be available for eligible patients.

Cost Reduction Strategies

Pill splitting for medications that come in higher strengths can reduce costs when medically appropriate and safe.

90-day supplies often cost less per dose than 30-day supplies and reduce pharmacy visits and copayments.

Generic alternatives should be considered when available and medically appropriate, with careful monitoring for effectiveness.

Combination medications may be more cost-effective than taking multiple separate drugs when appropriate combinations are available.

Emergency Medication Protocols

Having emergency medication plans helps you respond quickly to severe symptoms while avoiding dangerous delays in treatment.

Emergency Supply Planning

Essential medication identification involves determining which medications are critical for preventing dangerous symptoms versus those that primarily affect comfort or quality of life.

Emergency supplies should include at least a 72-hour supply of essential medications in a portable container that can be accessed quickly during crises.

Expiration date management ensures that emergency supplies remain effective and are rotated regularly to prevent degradation.

Storage considerations include temperature requirements, light sensitivity, and moisture protection for emergency medication supplies.

Crisis Intervention Protocols

MCAS emergency medications may include epinephrine auto-injectors, high-dose antihistamines, or corticosteroids for severe reactions.

POTS crisis management might require additional beta-blockers, fluid replacement solutions, or specific positioning and activity modifications.

Pain crisis protocols could include breakthrough pain medications, anti-inflammatory drugs, or muscle relaxants for severe EDS-related pain episodes.

Medical contact information should be readily available for accessing emergency care or consulting with your medical team during crises.

Family and Caregiver Training

Medication administration training helps family members assist with emergency medications when you're unable to manage them yourself.

Symptom recognition education enables caregivers to identify situations that require emergency medication use or medical attention.

Emergency contact protocols ensure that caregivers know when and how to contact medical providers or emergency services.

Documentation systems help caregivers communicate effectively with medical providers about your medication use and symptom management during emergencies.

Rachel's pharmacy consultation, described at the beginning of this section, resulted in a completely restructured medication schedule that improved her symptom control while reducing side effects. The key was viewing her medications as an orchestra that needed coordination rather than individual instruments playing separately.

This orchestrated approach to medication management requires ongoing attention and adjustment as your conditions change, new medications are added, or side effects develop. Success comes from understanding how each medication fits into your overall treatment symphony and working with your healthcare team to conduct that symphony effectively.

Harmonizing Your Treatment Symphony

Medication management for trifecta patients requires the precision of a conductor and the flexibility of a jazz musician. You must coordinate multiple therapeutic interventions while adapting to the daily variations and unexpected changes that characterize chronic illness.

The relationships you build with pharmacists, physicians, and other healthcare providers create the support network that enables safe and effective medication management. These partnerships become even more important as your medication regimen evolves over time.

Moving forward, your optimized medication regimen provides the foundation for exploring additional therapeutic approaches covered in the next section. Conventional medications work most effectively when complemented by evidence-based integrative therapies that address aspects of health that drugs alone cannot manage.

Core Medication Management Principles

- Drug class understanding helps predict interactions and optimize timing for maximum therapeutic benefit

- Interaction awareness goes beyond simple incompatibility to include absorption, metabolism, and effectiveness relationships

- Strategic timing coordination aligns peak medication effects with symptom patterns and daily activities

- Side effect recognition distinguishes medication effects from disease symptoms through careful observation and tracking

- Pharmacy partnerships provide expert guidance for complex medication regimens and optimization opportunities

- Generic versus brand decisions require individual assessment of effectiveness, tolerability, and cost factors

- Travel planning ensures medication access and compliance despite schedule disruptions and regulatory requirements

- Cost management strategies reduce financial barriers to necessary medications through insurance optimization and assistance programs

Chapter 9: Integrative Approaches

Evidence-Based Complementary Therapies

The acupuncture needles formed a precise constellation across Elena's back as Dr. Chen adjusted the final placement with the focused attention of an artist perfecting a masterpiece. "This point," she explained, gently tapping a needle near Elena's spine, "traditionally supports kidney yang energy, but from a Western perspective, it may help regulate your autonomic nervous system." Elena had been skeptical about combining traditional Chinese medicine with her conventional POTS treatment, but six months of integrated care had produced improvements that neither approach had achieved alone.

Elena's experience reflects the growing recognition that chronic illness often requires therapeutic approaches beyond conventional medicine. While medications form the backbone of trifecta treatment, they don't address all aspects of these complex conditions. Chronic stress, nervous system dysregulation, tissue health, and overall resilience often require interventions that work through different mechanisms than pharmaceutical treatments.

The challenge lies in separating evidence-based complementary therapies from unproven treatments that promise miraculous cures. The internet overflows with testimonials about supplements, devices, and treatments that supposedly cure chronic illness, but most lack scientific support and some can be dangerous when combined with conventional treatments.

Success requires a systematic approach that evaluates complementary therapies based on scientific evidence, safety profiles, and potential interactions with conventional treatments. The goal isn't to replace conventional medicine but to enhance it with interventions that address aspects of health that medications alone cannot manage.

Supplement Science and Evidence-Based Selection

Supplement use among chronic illness patients approaches 80%, but most people choose supplements based on marketing claims rather than scientific evidence. Understanding how to evaluate supplement research helps you make informed decisions about which products might benefit your specific conditions.

Research Quality Assessment

Peer-reviewed studies provide the gold standard for supplement evidence, but the quality of these studies varies dramatically. Look for randomized controlled trials with adequate sample sizes, appropriate control groups, and relevant outcome measures (26).

Systematic reviews and meta-analyses provide higher-level evidence by analyzing multiple studies on the same intervention. These reviews can identify consistent benefits across different study populations and help assess overall evidence quality.

Study population relevance affects how results apply to your situation. Studies conducted in healthy populations may not translate to people with chronic illness, while studies in specific patient populations provide more relevant evidence.

Funding sources can introduce bias in supplement research. Industry-funded studies are more likely to report positive results than independent research, though industry funding doesn't automatically invalidate findings.

Publication bias affects supplement research because positive results are more likely to be published than negative results, creating an overly optimistic view of supplement effectiveness.

Supplement Categories with Evidence

Omega-3 fatty acids show consistent evidence for anti-inflammatory effects and may help with cardiovascular health, cognitive function, and mood regulation. EPA and DHA from fish oil provide the most research support, with typical therapeutic doses ranging from 1-3 grams daily (27).

Quality matters significantly for omega-3 supplements because rancid oils can be pro-inflammatory. Look for products with third-party testing for purity and freshness, and store supplements properly to prevent oxidation.

Magnesium deficiency is common in chronic illness and supplementation may help with muscle cramps, sleep quality, and nervous system function. Magnesium glycinate and magnesium malate tend to be better absorbed and less likely to cause digestive upset than magnesium oxide (28).

Dosing typically ranges from 200-400mg daily, but some patients may need higher doses under medical supervision. Start with lower doses and increase gradually to assess tolerance.

Vitamin D deficiency affects up to 80% of people with chronic illness and supplementation may improve immune function, bone health, and mood. Target blood levels of 40-60 ng/mL rather than just avoiding deficiency (29).

Dosing requirements vary significantly based on baseline levels, body weight, and absorption factors. Regular monitoring helps ensure appropriate dosing and prevents toxicity from excessive supplementation.

Coenzyme Q10 supports cellular energy production and may help with fatigue and exercise tolerance. The ubiquinol form may be better absorbed than ubiquinone, particularly in people with digestive issues (30).

Typical doses range from 100-300mg daily, taken with fat-containing meals to improve absorption. Benefits may take several months to become apparent.

MCAS-Specific Supplementation

Natural antihistamines like quercetin may provide mast cell stabilizing effects and reduce histamine release. Quercetin works best when combined with bromelain for enhanced absorption (31).

Dosing typically ranges from 500-1000mg twice daily, taken away from meals. Start with lower doses to assess tolerance because some people react to quercetin despite its antihistamine properties.

Vitamin C supports histamine metabolism and may help reduce overall histamine load. High doses (1000-3000mg daily) may provide antihistamine effects, but start with lower doses and increase gradually (32).

Buffered forms or calcium ascorbate may be better tolerated than ascorbic acid in people with sensitive digestive systems.

DAO enzyme supplements help break down dietary histamine and may allow greater food variety for people with histamine intolerance. Take 1-2 capsules before meals containing moderate-histamine foods (33).

Effectiveness varies significantly between individuals, and these supplements work only for dietary histamine, not endogenous histamine production.

POTS-Targeted Supplements

Electrolyte supplements help maintain blood volume and improve circulation when formulated with appropriate ratios of sodium, potassium, and magnesium. Avoid products with artificial colors and flavors that might trigger MCAS reactions.

Commercial electrolyte products often contain inadequate sodium for POTS patients. Custom formulations or multiple products may be needed to achieve therapeutic sodium levels.

Licorice root (deglycyrrhizinated form) may support blood pressure regulation through effects on aldosterone activity. Use DGL forms to avoid blood pressure elevation in sensitive individuals (34).

Monitor blood pressure regularly if using licorice supplements because effects can vary significantly between individuals.

Iron supplementation helps if deficiency is present because iron deficiency can worsen POTS symptoms. However, iron supplements can trigger digestive symptoms and MCAS reactions in some patients (35).

Use chelated forms like iron bisglycinate for better absorption and fewer side effects. Take with vitamin C and avoid taking with calcium or tea.

Mind-Body Interventions for Nervous System Regulation

Chronic stress and autonomic dysfunction create cycles where physical symptoms worsen stress, which then worsens physical symptoms. Mind-body interventions can break these cycles by directly affecting nervous system function and stress response patterns.

Meditation and Mindfulness Practices

Mindfulness-based stress reduction (MBSR) shows consistent evidence for reducing pain, improving mood, and supporting immune function in chronic illness. The practice involves focusing attention on present-moment experiences without judgment (36).

Research specifically in POTS patients shows that mindfulness practices can improve heart rate variability and reduce symptom severity. Even short daily practices of 10-20 minutes can provide measurable benefits.

Meditation techniques vary widely, and finding approaches that work for your personality and limitations is important. Body scan meditations may be challenging for people with chronic pain, while breathing-focused practices might trigger anxiety in some individuals.

Guided meditations through apps or recordings can provide structure for beginners and help maintain consistent practice during difficult periods.

Progressive muscle relaxation involves systematically tensing and relaxing muscle groups to reduce physical tension and promote relaxation responses. This technique can be particularly helpful for EDS patients who experience chronic muscle tension (37).

Modified versions avoid excessive stretching or joint stress while still providing relaxation benefits. Focus on gentle muscle contractions rather than maximum tension.

Breathing Techniques for Autonomic Balance

Diaphragmatic breathing activates the parasympathetic nervous system and can help regulate heart rate variability in POTS patients. This technique involves breathing deeply into the belly rather than the chest (38).

Practice starts with short sessions of 2-3 minutes and gradually increases as comfort and skill develop. Some people initially feel lightheaded or anxious with deep breathing practices.

Box breathing involves equal counts for inhalation, holding, exhalation, and holding again. A common pattern is 4 counts for each phase, but adjust timing based on comfort and lung capacity.

This technique can be particularly helpful for managing anxiety and preparing for challenging activities or medical appointments.

Coherent breathing at 5-6 breaths per minute can improve heart rate variability and autonomic balance. This slower breathing rate requires practice but can provide significant benefits for POTS symptoms (39).

Use apps or devices that provide visual or auditory pacing to maintain consistent breathing rates during practice sessions.

Biofeedback and Technology-Assisted Interventions

Heart rate variability (HRV) biofeedback teaches patients to control autonomic nervous system responses through real-time feedback about heart rhythm patterns. This intervention shows particular promise for POTS management (40).

Training typically involves 10-20 sessions with a qualified practitioner, followed by home practice using HRV devices or apps. Improvements may continue for months after training completion.

EMG biofeedback helps patients learn to control muscle tension patterns that contribute to pain and dysfunction. This can be particularly helpful for EDS patients who develop compensatory muscle tension.

Temperature biofeedback teaches relaxation responses through awareness of skin temperature changes that reflect blood flow and nervous system activity.

Neurofeedback involves training brain wave patterns associated with relaxation, focus, or other desired states. While research is limited, some patients report benefits for cognitive symptoms and sleep quality.

Yoga and Tai Chi Adaptations

Therapeutic yoga focuses on gentle movements, breathing practices, and relaxation rather than achieving challenging poses. Chair yoga or supported positions can accommodate mobility limitations (41).

Avoid excessive stretching or end-range positions that might worsen joint hypermobility in EDS patients. Focus on strengthening and stability rather than increasing flexibility.

Tai chi provides gentle movement therapy that can improve balance, reduce fall risk, and support stress management. The slow, controlled movements are generally safe for people with chronic illness (42).

Modified versions can be performed seated or with support to accommodate different ability levels and symptoms.

Yin yoga uses supported positions held for longer periods to promote relaxation without requiring strength or flexibility. Props like bolsters and blocks provide support and comfort.

Physical Therapies and Manual Treatments

Hands-on therapies can address tissue health, circulation, and nervous system function through mechanisms that complement conventional medical treatments. However, finding practitioners who understand chronic illness limitations is essential for safety and effectiveness.

Massage Therapy Considerations

Therapeutic massage can improve circulation, reduce muscle tension, and support stress management when performed by therapists who understand chronic illness limitations. However, aggressive massage can worsen symptoms in sensitive patients (43).

Pressure tolerance varies significantly in chronic illness patients. Start with very light pressure and communicate constantly with therapists about comfort levels.

Lymphatic drainage massage may help with fluid retention and circulation issues common in POTS patients. This specialized technique requires training in lymphatic system anatomy and physiology.

Trigger point therapy can address specific areas of muscle tension and dysfunction, but must be performed carefully in hypermobile patients to avoid joint injury.

Contraindications include active inflammation, severe autonomic instability, or acute injury. Some patients experience temporary symptom worsening after massage before noticing benefits.

Acupuncture for Trifecta Conditions

Traditional acupuncture shows evidence for pain management, nausea reduction, and stress relief that may benefit trifecta patients. Research specifically in POTS patients suggests improvements in heart rate variability and symptom severity (44).

Point selection should be individualized based on your specific symptoms and constitution. Practitioners trained in both traditional Chinese medicine and Western medical concepts may provide more integrated care.

Electroacupuncture combines traditional needle placement with electrical stimulation and may provide enhanced effects for pain and autonomic symptoms.

Auricular (ear) acupuncture provides a portable option that can be maintained between full treatments. Small seeds or semi-permanent needles allow continuous stimulation of specific points.

Safety considerations include needle sterility, practitioner training, and awareness of your bleeding tendencies or immune sensitivities. Some patients with MCAS may react to needle materials or topical preparations used during treatment.

Craniosacral Therapy and Osteopathic Approaches

Craniosacral therapy involves gentle manipulation of skull bones and spinal tissues to improve cerebrospinal fluid flow and nervous system function. While research is limited, some patients report improvements in headaches and autonomic symptoms (45).

Gentle techniques are essential for EDS patients whose tissues may be more fragile and prone to injury from manipulation. Practitioners should understand hypermobility disorders before treating these patients.

Osteopathic manipulative treatment (OMT) focuses on improving tissue mobility and function through various manual techniques. Osteopathic physicians can integrate these approaches with conventional medical care.

Visceral manipulation addresses restrictions in organ movement and may help with digestive symptoms common in trifecta patients.

Contraindications include acute injury, severe instability, or recent surgery. Some techniques may not be appropriate for patients with vascular EDS or other connective tissue disorders with fragility.

Chiropractic Considerations for EDS

Spinal manipulation requires extreme caution in EDS patients due to ligament laxity and potential for injury. High-velocity, low-amplitude adjustments may be contraindicated in some patients.

Gentle mobilization techniques may be safer alternatives that can still provide benefits for joint function and pain management.

Upper cervical instability is a particular concern in EDS patients and requires specialized evaluation before any neck manipulation.

Imaging studies may be needed before chiropractic treatment to identify structural abnormalities or instabilities that would contraindicate manipulation.

Activity-based treatments like exercises and ergonomic advice may provide more benefits than hands-on manipulation for many EDS patients.

Technology Aids and Medical Devices

Various devices can provide symptom relief, monitoring capabilities, and therapeutic benefits that complement other treatment approaches. Understanding which devices have evidence support helps guide investment decisions.

TENS Units and Electrical Stimulation

Transcutaneous electrical nerve stimulation (TENS) can provide pain relief through gate control mechanisms that block pain signals to the brain. Units are available for home use and may help with localized EDS-related pain (46).

Electrode placement affects effectiveness and requires some experimentation to find optimal positions for your specific pain patterns. Start with manufacturer recommendations and adjust based on response.

Stimulation parameters including frequency, intensity, and duration can be adjusted for different types of pain. Higher frequencies may work better for acute pain, while lower frequencies might help with chronic pain.

Contraindications include pacemakers, pregnancy, and placement over areas of decreased sensation. Some patients with MCAS may react to electrode adhesives.

Interferential current therapy uses higher frequency electrical stimulation that may penetrate deeper tissues and provide longer-lasting pain relief than traditional TENS units.

Compression Garments and Devices

Graduated compression stockings provide mechanical support for circulation and can significantly improve POTS symptoms by preventing blood pooling in the legs. Compression levels of 20-30 mmHg are typically recommended (47).

Proper fitting is essential for effectiveness and comfort. Professional fitting ensures appropriate size and compression level for your specific needs.

Abdominal binders can help some POTS patients by compressing abdominal blood vessels and improving venous return. These should be used under medical supervision.

Compression garments for other body areas may help with swelling, joint support, or proprioceptive awareness in EDS patients.

Pneumatic compression devices provide intermittent compression that may help with circulation and lymphatic drainage. These are typically used for specific medical conditions under physician guidance.

Temperature and Environmental Devices

Cooling vests and products can help prevent overheating that triggers POTS and MCAS symptoms. Various designs are available from simple cooling towels to sophisticated vest systems.

Heating pads and devices may help with EDS-related muscle tension and joint pain, but must be used carefully to avoid burns in patients with decreased sensation.

Air purifiers with HEPA filtration can reduce environmental triggers for MCAS patients. Choose units appropriate for room size and look for low ozone production.

Humidifiers and dehumidifiers help maintain optimal humidity levels that may reduce respiratory symptoms and improve comfort.

White noise machines or apps can improve sleep quality by masking environmental sounds that might trigger stress responses or prevent deep sleep.

Monitoring and Biofeedback Devices

Heart rate monitors provide objective data about POTS symptoms and exercise responses. Chest strap monitors typically provide more accurate data than wrist-based devices during activity.

Blood pressure monitors for home use help track treatment effectiveness and identify concerning changes that need medical attention. Choose validated devices appropriate for your arm size.

Sleep tracking devices can provide insights into sleep quality and patterns that affect symptom management. While not as accurate as professional sleep studies, they can identify trends and responses to interventions.

Continuous glucose monitors may be helpful for patients who experience blood sugar fluctuations that affect their symptoms, even if they don't have diabetes.

Pulse oximeters measure oxygen saturation and can help identify breathing issues that might contribute to symptoms or indicate need for medical attention.

Provider Vetting and Integration

Finding qualified complementary practitioners who understand chronic illness requires research and careful evaluation. The integration of these providers with your conventional medical team requires communication and coordination.

Practitioner Qualification Assessment

Educational background should include formal training from accredited institutions relevant to their practice area. Licensure requirements vary by state and profession.

Chronic illness experience indicates practitioners who understand the special considerations and limitations of people with complex medical conditions.

Continuing education demonstrates commitment to staying current with research and best practices in their field.

Professional associations and certifications provide additional quality indicators and may offer complaint resolution processes.

Patient references from others with similar conditions can provide insights into practitioner effectiveness and communication styles.

Red Flags in Alternative Medicine

Cure claims should be viewed with extreme skepticism because chronic illnesses like trifecta conditions are not curable through any known interventions.

Expensive upfront payment requirements for extensive treatment packages may indicate practitioners more interested in profit than patient care.

Recommendations to stop conventional treatments without medical supervision can be dangerous and indicate practitioners who don't understand the serious nature of your conditions.

Unproven diagnostic methods like live blood analysis or applied kinesiology lack scientific support and may lead to inappropriate treatments.

Supplement sales pressure suggests potential conflicts of interest that may influence treatment recommendations.

Communication with Conventional Providers

Disclosure of all complementary treatments to your conventional medical team prevents dangerous interactions and ensures coordinated care.

Treatment goal alignment helps ensure that complementary and conventional treatments work toward the same objectives rather than at cross-purposes.

Progress monitoring should include both conventional medical markers and complementary therapy outcomes to assess overall treatment effectiveness.

Interaction awareness requires communication about all interventions because even "natural" treatments can interact with medications or affect medical conditions.

Emergency protocols should include information about complementary treatments that might affect emergency care decisions.

DIY Techniques and Self-Administration

Many effective complementary therapies can be learned and practiced at home, providing cost-effective options for ongoing symptom management.

Self-Massage and Pressure Point Techniques

Trigger point self-release using tennis balls, foam rollers, or specialized tools can help manage muscle tension and pain between professional treatments.

Pressure application should be gentle and gradual, particularly in EDS patients whose tissues may be more fragile than normal.

Self-massage techniques for hands, feet, and accessible areas can improve circulation and provide stress relief during daily activities.

Lymphatic drainage techniques can be learned for self-administration to help with fluid retention and circulation issues.

Breathing and Relaxation Protocols

Progressive muscle relaxation scripts can be learned and practiced independently using audio guides or written instructions.

Breathing exercise progression starts with simple techniques and gradually introduces more advanced practices as skill and comfort develop.

Meditation apps provide guided sessions appropriate for different experience levels and time constraints.

Visualization techniques can be practiced anywhere and may help with pain management, anxiety, and sleep preparation.

Stress Management Tools

Journaling practices can help identify stress patterns and triggers while providing emotional outlet and processing opportunities.

Time management strategies help reduce stress from overcommitment and poor planning that can worsen chronic illness symptoms.

Boundary setting skills help protect energy and reduce stress from excessive demands or unsuitable social situations.

Problem-solving frameworks provide structured approaches to addressing chronic illness challenges and reducing associated stress.

Cost-Benefit Analysis and Prioritization

Limited financial resources require strategic decisions about which complementary therapies provide the best value for your specific needs and circumstances.

Evidence-Based Prioritization

Research strength should guide initial investments in complementary therapies. Interventions with strong evidence deserve higher priority than those with limited research support.

Safety profiles affect cost-benefit calculations because therapies with higher risk of adverse effects require more careful monitoring and may create additional medical costs.

Potential for self-administration makes some therapies more cost-effective over time because they don't require ongoing professional visits.

Integration with existing treatments may create synergistic effects that provide greater benefits than individual interventions alone.

Cost-Effectiveness Evaluation

Professional treatment costs include not just session fees but also travel time, energy expenditure, and potential time off work.

Equipment and supply costs for home-based interventions should be amortized over expected useful life to calculate true per-session costs.

Opportunity costs include other treatments or activities that can't be pursued due to financial or time limitations.

Insurance coverage varies widely for complementary therapies, but some services may be covered under certain circumstances or through flexible spending accounts.

Budget Planning Strategies

Phased implementation allows you to try one intervention at a time and assess benefits before adding additional treatments.

Seasonal planning may allow you to take advantage of provider promotions or budget for treatments during specific times of year.

Group classes or sessions often cost less than individual treatments while still providing many of the same benefits.

Combination packages from individual providers may offer cost savings compared to purchasing sessions individually.

Safety Considerations and Interaction Awareness

Complementary therapies can interact with conventional treatments or worsen underlying conditions if not used appropriately. Understanding these risks helps you make informed decisions about treatment combinations.

Supplement-Medication Interactions

Herb-drug interactions can affect medication metabolism, absorption, or effectiveness. St. John's wort, for example, can reduce the effectiveness of many medications by increasing liver enzyme activity (48).

Timing interactions occur when supplements affect the absorption of medications. Calcium and iron supplements can reduce absorption of certain antibiotics and thyroid medications.

Additive effects happen when supplements and medications affect the same physiological systems. Multiple blood-thinning supplements combined with anticoagulant medications can increase bleeding risk.

Monitoring requirements may increase when combining supplements with medications that require regular blood tests or other monitoring.

Physical Therapy Contraindications

Acute inflammation contraindicated many hands-on therapies that might worsen tissue damage or delay healing.

Bleeding disorders or anticoagulant medications may increase risk of bruising or bleeding from massage or manipulation.

Joint instability in EDS patients requires modified techniques and careful practitioner selection to avoid injury.

Autonomic instability may make some positioning or treatment approaches problematic for POTS patients.

Immune System Considerations

Immune suppression from medications or disease processes may increase infection risk from acupuncture needles or other invasive interventions.

MCAS patients may react unpredictably to topical preparations, massage oils, or other products used during complementary treatments.

Stress from new treatments or travel to appointments can trigger symptom flares in sensitive individuals.

Emergency Preparedness

Adverse reaction protocols should be established before starting new treatments, particularly for patients with histories of severe reactions.

Emergency contact information for both conventional and complementary providers ensures appropriate response to problems.

Treatment discontinuation plans help patients safely stop complementary therapies if problems develop or if they interfere with conventional treatments.

Elena's success with integrated acupuncture and conventional POTS treatment, described at the beginning of this section, demonstrates the potential for complementary therapies to enhance conventional care. Her improvement required finding a qualified acupuncturist who understood autonomic dysfunction and was willing to communicate with her conventional medical team.

The key to successful integration lies in evidence-based selection, qualified practitioners, and clear communication between all members of your healthcare team. Complementary therapies work best when they're viewed as part of a coordinated treatment approach rather than alternatives to conventional care.

Building Your Integrative Treatment Plan

Successful integration of complementary therapies requires systematic evaluation, careful planning, and ongoing monitoring of results. The goal is enhancing your conventional treatment rather than replacing it with unproven alternatives.

The relationships you build with qualified complementary practitioners become part of your extended healthcare team, providing additional perspectives and treatment options for managing complex chronic conditions.

Moving forward, the integrative approaches you've learned can provide additional tools for managing the crisis situations and emergency protocols covered in the next section. Mind-body techniques, in particular, can be valuable during acute symptom flares when conventional medications may not be sufficient.

Essential Principles for Integrative Care

- Evidence-based supplement selection prioritizes interventions with research support over marketing claims or testimonials

- Mind-body interventions directly affect nervous system function and can break cycles of stress and symptom escalation

- Physical therapies require practitioners who understand chronic illness limitations and can modify treatments appropriately

- Technology aids and devices can provide objective monitoring and therapeutic benefits when selected based on evidence

- Provider vetting ensures that complementary practitioners have appropriate training and understand chronic illness complexities

- DIY techniques provide cost-effective options for ongoing symptom management between professional treatments

- Cost-benefit analysis helps prioritize limited resources toward interventions with the strongest evidence and best fit for individual needs

- Safety considerations prevent harmful interactions between complementary and conventional treatments

Chapter 10: Crisis Management

The emergency room physician looked puzzled as she reviewed Amanda's vital signs for the third time. Heart rate 145, blood pressure 90/60, temperature normal, oxygen saturation perfect. "Your heart rate is quite elevated," she said, "but all your other tests are normal. Are you having anxiety about something?" Amanda wanted to scream. This was exactly what she'd feared—another medical professional who didn't understand that her racing heart, flushed skin, and overwhelming fatigue weren't anxiety but a trifecta flare that required specific interventions, not dismissive reassurance.

Amanda's emergency department experience represents one of the most challenging aspects of living with POTS, MCAS, and EDS—managing acute symptom flares and true medical emergencies in a healthcare system that often doesn't recognize these conditions. Crisis situations can develop rapidly and unpredictably, leaving patients and families scrambling to get appropriate care while navigating medical professionals who may be unfamiliar with trifecta conditions.

The complexity increases because trifecta patients can experience true medical emergencies that require immediate intervention, symptom flares that need urgent but non-emergency care, and chronic symptom variations that feel alarming but don't require immediate medical attention. Distinguishing between these scenarios while managing the stress and symptoms of acute illness requires preparation, knowledge, and clear protocols.

Successful crisis management begins long before emergencies occur. It requires developing early warning systems, creating action plans for different scenarios, educating family members and advocates, and establishing relationships with medical providers who understand your conditions. Most importantly, it requires learning to navigate emergency medical care while maintaining your dignity and ensuring appropriate treatment.

Recognizing Early Warning Signs

Early intervention often prevents minor symptom changes from escalating into major crises. Understanding your personal warning signs and having protocols for responding to them can significantly reduce the frequency and severity of acute episodes.

Individual Pattern Recognition

Baseline establishment helps you recognize when symptoms are truly worse than usual versus part of normal fluctuations. Your "normal bad day" may look alarming to others but not require emergency intervention, while subtle changes from your baseline might indicate developing crises.

Tracking unusual combinations of symptoms often provides earlier warning than waiting for severe individual symptoms. You might notice that mild nausea combined with slight increase in heart rate and unusual fatigue predicts a larger flare within 12-24 hours.

Environmental trigger awareness helps identify external factors that might precipitate crises. Changes in weather, exposure to allergens, emotional stress, or disruptions in routine can all trigger symptom escalation in sensitive individuals.

Medication effectiveness changes may signal developing problems. If medications that usually provide reliable symptom control become less effective, this often indicates that intervention may be needed before symptoms worsen significantly.

Prodromal Symptom Identification

Pre-flare symptoms vary between individuals but often follow consistent patterns for each person. Some patients experience increased brain fog, mood changes, or sleep disturbances 24-48 hours before major symptom episodes.

Autonomic warning signs in POTS patients might include increased orthostatic symptoms, temperature regulation problems, or digestive changes that indicate autonomic nervous system destabilization.

MCAS prodromal symptoms often include increased sensitivity to environmental triggers, mild skin reactions, or digestive symptoms that precede more severe reactions.

EDS warning signs might include increased joint pain, muscle tension, or subluxations that indicate overall connective tissue stress that could lead to more significant problems.

Sleep pattern changes frequently precede symptom flares across all three conditions. Difficulty falling asleep, frequent awakening, or non-restorative sleep often signals developing problems.

Stress and Trigger Accumulation

Threshold recognition helps you understand when multiple minor stressors combine to create risk for major symptoms. You might tolerate individual triggers well but experience severe symptoms when several occur simultaneously.

Cumulative stress assessment includes physical, emotional, and environmental stressors that may not seem directly related to your medical conditions but can trigger symptom escalation.

Recovery debt occurs when you haven't fully recovered from previous symptom episodes before new stressors occur. This creates a downward spiral where each episode makes you more vulnerable to the next.

Life event timing affects your vulnerability to symptom flares. Moving, job changes, family stress, or other major life events can increase your risk for several weeks or months.

Case Study: Early Intervention Success

Maria learned to recognize her pre-flare pattern after tracking symptoms for several months. She noticed that irritability combined with mild digestive upset and slightly elevated resting heart rate predicted major POTS episodes within 24-36 hours.

When these warning signs appeared, Maria implemented her early intervention protocol. She increased fluid and salt intake, cleared her schedule for rest, took additional antihistamines, and arranged for help with household responsibilities.

This early intervention reduced her emergency department visits from once monthly to twice yearly and significantly decreased the severity of symptoms when flares did occur.

Her family learned to recognize her warning signs and support her intervention efforts.

Home Management Protocols

Effective home management can resolve many symptom flares without requiring medical attention while providing clear criteria for when professional care is needed.

POTS Crisis Management

Position management forms the foundation of POTS crisis intervention. Lying down with legs elevated often provides immediate symptom relief by improving venous return and reducing orthostatic stress.

Graduated position changes help prevent symptom escalation when getting up is necessary. Move from lying to sitting to standing slowly, pausing at each position to allow cardiovascular adjustment.

Hydration protocols for POTS flares involve immediate fluid replacement with electrolyte solutions rather than plain water. Aim for 16-24 ounces of fluid over 30-60 minutes if tolerated.

Activity restriction prevents symptom escalation during acute episodes. Avoid unnecessary standing, walking, or exertion until symptoms stabilize, typically 2-4 hours for mild episodes.

Temperature management includes avoiding heat exposure that can worsen vasodilation and orthostatic intolerance. Cool environments and cooling methods may provide symptom relief.

Medication adjustments might include additional doses of prescribed medications if specifically approved by your medical team for crisis situations.

MCAS Reaction Protocols

Trigger removal represents the first priority when possible MCAS triggers can be identified and eliminated. Move away from environmental triggers, discontinue suspect foods or medications, and reduce sensory stimulation.

Antihistamine escalation follows predetermined protocols established with your medical team. This might involve taking additional doses of current medications or adding different types of antihistamines.

Epinephrine administration becomes necessary for severe reactions involving breathing difficulties, severe swelling, or cardiovascular symptoms. Follow your emergency action plan for epinephrine use and always seek emergency care after administration (49).

Symptom monitoring includes tracking reaction progression to determine if home management is effective or if emergency care is needed. Document timing, triggers, symptoms, and interventions.

Cool down measures help manage flushing and overheating that accompany many MCAS reactions. Cool cloths, cool environments, and removal of restrictive clothing may provide relief.

EDS Pain and Injury Management

Joint protection involves immediate immobilization of injured or unstable joints using splints, braces, or supportive positioning. Avoid movement that causes sharp pain or instability.

Subluxation reduction for patients trained in self-reduction techniques, but never attempt reduction of joints you haven't been trained to manage or that seem severely displaced.

Pain management follows a stepwise approach using medications and non-pharmacological methods as predetermined with your medical team. Ice, heat, positioning, and gentle movement may help with some types of pain.

Swelling control includes elevation of affected areas and gentle compression if appropriate. Avoid tight compression that might impair circulation.

Activity modification prevents further injury while allowing safe movement. Use assistive devices, modify tasks, or arrange help with activities that stress injured areas.

Documentation for Medical Care

Crisis tracking provides essential information for medical providers and helps identify patterns that might guide prevention strategies. Record symptom onset, severity, triggers, interventions, and outcomes.

Photo documentation of visible symptoms like rashes, swelling, or joint positions can provide valuable information for medical providers, especially if symptoms resolve before evaluation.

Vital sign monitoring using home devices provides objective data that supports your symptom reports. Blood pressure, heart rate, and temperature measurements can guide treatment decisions.

Treatment response documentation shows medical providers which interventions have been tried and their effectiveness, preventing repetition of ineffective treatments.

Emergency Department Navigation

Emergency departments are designed for acute, life-threatening conditions and may not be well-equipped to handle chronic illness flares. Successful navigation requires preparation, clear communication, and realistic expectations.

Preparation for Emergency Care

Emergency information cards provide quick reference for medical staff unfamiliar with your conditions. Include current medications, known allergies, emergency contacts, and specific medical needs.

Medical summary letters from your physician explain your conditions, typical symptoms, and recommended treatments. These letters can significantly improve emergency care quality.

Current medication lists should include dosages, timing, and specific instructions for emergency situations. Include both prescription and over-the-counter medications.

Emergency contact information for your medical team helps emergency providers consult with physicians familiar with your conditions and treatment needs.

Insurance and identification documents prevent delays in care and ensure that emergency treatment is properly documented and billed.

Communication Strategies

Clear symptom description focuses on objective, measurable symptoms rather than subjective descriptions that might be misinterpreted. "Heart rate 150 when standing" is more helpful than "feeling funny."

Treatment history explanation helps emergency providers understand what has been tried and what might be effective. Bring lists of medications that have helped or caused problems in the past.

Diagnostic awareness prevents unnecessary testing while ensuring that serious conditions are appropriately evaluated. Know which symptoms require immediate evaluation versus those that are typical for your conditions.

Family advocate coordination ensures that someone can speak for you if symptoms affect your ability to communicate clearly. Designate a family member or friend as your medical advocate.

Common Emergency Department Challenges

Symptom minimization occurs when emergency staff unfamiliar with your conditions assume symptoms are less serious than they are. Objective data like vital signs can help support your reports.

Inappropriate discharge may occur when emergency providers don't understand the serious nature of trifecta conditions or assume symptoms are psychological.

Medication restrictions might prevent you from receiving medications that have been effective in the past. Bring documentation from your physicians about specific medication needs.

Testing limitations in emergency departments may not include specialized tests needed to evaluate your conditions appropriately.

Crisis Prevention Strategies

Preventing crises is more effective than managing them after they occur. Lifestyle modifications and proactive management can significantly reduce the frequency and severity of acute episodes.

Lifestyle Stability Measures

Routine maintenance helps prevent the disruptions that can trigger symptom flares. Consistent sleep schedules, meal timing, and daily activities support physiological stability.

Stress management becomes particularly important for preventing crises because stress often triggers symptom escalation across all three conditions.

Environmental control includes managing known triggers in your home and work environments. Air quality, temperature, allergen exposure, and noise levels all affect symptom stability.

Social support systems provide assistance during stressful periods and help with practical needs that might otherwise trigger symptom flares.

Medical Management Optimization

Medication compliance prevents symptom rebound that can occur when treatments are missed or taken inconsistently.

Regular medical follow-up helps identify developing problems before they become crises and allows for proactive treatment adjustments.

Laboratory monitoring catches problems like electrolyte imbalances or vitamin deficiencies that might predispose to symptom flares.

Vaccination status maintenance prevents infections that can trigger severe symptom exacerbations in people with chronic illness.

Activity and Energy Management

Pacing strategies prevent the overexertion that commonly triggers symptom flares. Learn to recognize your energy limits and plan activities accordingly.

Recovery time planning includes building adequate rest periods into your schedule, particularly after demanding activities or stressful events.

Warning sign response protocols help you implement preventive measures when early symptoms appear, potentially preventing full crisis development.

Emergency Action Plans

Written protocols for different emergency scenarios help you and your family respond quickly and appropriately to crisis situations while reducing panic and confusion.

MCAS Emergency Protocols

Anaphylaxis recognition and response requires understanding the signs of severe allergic reactions and having clear protocols for epinephrine administration and emergency medical care (50).

Epinephrine auto-injectors should be available in multiple locations and all family members should know how to use them. Replace expired devices and ensure that backup devices are available.

Emergency medication protocols include specific instructions for antihistamine dosing, corticosteroid use if prescribed, and other medications that might be helpful during severe reactions.

Emergency contact procedures ensure rapid access to emergency medical services and notification of your medical team about severe reactions.

POTS Emergency Scenarios

Severe orthostatic intolerance may require emergency medical evaluation when home management fails to provide symptom relief or when symptoms suggest serious complications.

Syncope (fainting) protocols include safety measures to prevent injury and criteria for seeking emergency care based on frequency, duration, or associated symptoms.

Cardiac symptom evaluation helps distinguish between POTS-related symptoms and potential cardiac emergencies that require immediate medical attention.

Dehydration recognition and response includes understanding when fluid losses or poor intake require medical intervention rather than home management.

EDS Emergency Situations

Major joint dislocations require emergency medical attention, particularly for hips, shoulders, or any joint that can't be safely reduced or that has associated numbness or circulation problems.

Suspected fractures need emergency evaluation because EDS patients may have increased fracture risk and unusual fracture patterns.

Vascular complications, while rare, can be life-threatening in certain EDS types and require immediate emergency medical attention.

Severe pain that doesn't respond to usual management may indicate complications that require medical evaluation.

Hospital Preparation and Advocacy

Hospital stays require special preparation for trifecta patients because inpatient staff may be unfamiliar with these conditions and their management requirements.

Hospital Bag Essentials

Medical documentation should include current medication lists, physician contact information, medical summaries, and any special equipment or supplies you might need.

Personal comfort items help manage the stress of hospitalization and provide familiar objects that support emotional well-being during difficult periods.

Medication supplies ensure continuity of treatment if hospital formularies don't include your specific medications or if you need higher doses than typically stocked.

Communication tools include phone chargers, contact lists, and any adaptive equipment you use for communication if illness affects your ability to speak clearly.

Staff Education Strategies

Condition explanation materials help hospital staff understand your conditions and their implications for care. Bring printed materials from patient organizations or your physicians.

Treatment preference communication ensures that hospital staff understand which interventions have been helpful or harmful in the past.

Monitoring requirement explanation helps nursing staff understand which vital signs and symptoms need special attention in trifecta patients.

Discharge planning coordination ensures that your outpatient medical team is involved in hospital discharge planning and that appropriate follow-up is arranged.

Insurance and Legal Considerations

Advanced directives ensure that your treatment preferences are known if you become unable to communicate them during severe illness.

Medical power of attorney designation allows trusted individuals to make medical decisions on your behalf if necessary.

Insurance authorization may be needed for certain treatments or extended stays, and having emergency contact information for your insurance company can prevent delays.

Privacy preferences should be communicated regarding who can receive information about your care and who can visit during hospitalization.

Recovery Protocols

Recovery from acute episodes often takes longer than the acute phase and requires specific strategies to prevent rebound symptoms and support healing.

Immediate Post-Crisis Care

Activity restriction continues during early recovery to prevent symptom rebound. Gradually increase activity levels based on symptom tolerance rather than predetermined timelines.

Medication continuation or adjustment may be needed during recovery, particularly if emergency treatments affected your usual medication regimen.

Symptom monitoring helps identify complications or slow recovery that might need medical attention.

Trigger avoidance becomes particularly important during recovery when your threshold for symptom recurrence may be lower than usual.

Long-term Recovery Planning

Rest and rehabilitation balance the need for recovery time with maintenance of function and prevention of deconditioning.

Gradual activity resumption follows structured progression that prevents overexertion while supporting return to baseline function.

Medical follow-up ensures that recovery is progressing appropriately and addresses any complications or concerns that develop.

Learning from Crisis Episodes

Episode analysis helps identify triggers, warning signs, and effective interventions that can improve future crisis management.

Protocol refinement based on experience helps optimize your emergency plans and improve outcomes during future episodes.

Prevention strategy adjustment may be needed if crisis episodes reveal gaps in your current management approach.

Amanda's emergency department experience, described at the beginning of this section, improved dramatically after she developed comprehensive crisis management protocols. She learned to bring documentation that helped emergency staff understand her conditions, practiced clear communication strategies, and established relationships with emergency physicians at her local hospital.

Crisis management for trifecta patients requires preparation, education, and advocacy skills that extend beyond medical knowledge. You become an expert in your own care while building systems that support you during vulnerable periods when illness may affect your ability to advocate for yourself.

Crisis as Learning Opportunity

Each crisis episode, while challenging, provides information that can improve your long-term management and reduce future emergency needs. The goal isn't to eliminate all crises but to minimize their frequency, severity, and impact on your life.

The crisis management skills you develop serve you beyond medical emergencies. They improve your confidence in managing chronic illness, your ability to advocate effectively, and your capacity to support others facing similar challenges.

Moving forward, the crisis prevention and management strategies you've learned provide the foundation for the long-term lifestyle integration approaches covered in upcoming sections. Effective crisis management creates the stability that makes planning for work, relationships, and life goals possible.

Core Crisis Management Elements

- Early warning sign recognition enables proactive intervention that can prevent minor symptoms from escalating into major crises

- Home management protocols provide structured approaches to treating symptom flares while maintaining clear criteria for seeking professional care

- Emergency department navigation requires preparation, clear communication, and realistic expectations about acute care capabilities

- Crisis prevention strategies focus on lifestyle stability, medical optimization, and proactive stress management

- Emergency action plans provide written protocols for different scenarios that reduce panic and ensure appropriate responses

- Hospital preparation includes documentation, advocacy strategies, and legal considerations for inpatient care

- Recovery protocols support healing while preventing rebound symptoms and supporting return to baseline function

- Learning from crises improves future management through analysis of triggers, warning signs, and effective interventions

Chapter 11: Professional Life Redesign

Career Success with Chronic Illness

The conference room fell silent as Katherine carefully chose her words during the quarterly review meeting. Her boss had just questioned why her productivity metrics looked different from her colleagues', and she faced a choice that countless professionals with chronic illness know well—reveal her POTS, MCAS, and EDS diagnoses to explain her modified work patterns, or continue managing in silence while her career prospects dimmed. Three years earlier, Katherine had been a rising star in marketing, working sixty-hour weeks and traveling constantly. Now, she needed a different approach to success—one that honored both her professional ambitions and her physical realities.

Katherine's dilemma represents the central challenge of professional life with chronic illness: how do you build a meaningful career when your body operates by different rules than the traditional workplace expects? The old model of career success—linear advancement, consistent high-energy output, and unlimited availability—simply doesn't work for people whose energy fluctuates, who need medical appointments, and who require environmental accommodations.

Yet career success remains possible when you understand your rights, develop strategic approaches to productivity, and learn to advocate for the accommodations that allow you to perform at your best. The key lies in redefining success on your terms while building the skills and relationships that support long-term professional growth.

210

Modern workplace trends actually favor many of the adaptations that chronic illness requires. Remote work has become mainstream, flexible schedules are increasingly common, and results-oriented cultures focus more on outcomes than hours logged. These changes create opportunities for people with chronic illness to thrive professionally in ways that weren't possible even a decade ago.

Understanding Workplace Accommodation Rights

The Americans with Disabilities Act (ADA) provides the legal framework that protects employees with chronic illness, but understanding your rights requires more than knowing the law exists. Effective advocacy requires specific knowledge about covered conditions, reasonable accommodations, and the interactive process that determines workplace modifications.

ADA Coverage and Qualifying Conditions

Disability definition under the ADA includes conditions that substantially limit major life activities, have a record of such impairment, or are regarded as having such impairment. POTS, MCAS, and EDS can all qualify as disabilities when they significantly affect major life activities like walking, standing, breathing, concentrating, or working (51).

Major life activities encompass both basic functions like breathing and walking, and major bodily functions including cardiovascular, immune, and musculoskeletal systems. Trifecta conditions often affect multiple systems, strengthening the case for ADA coverage.

Substantial limitation doesn't require complete inability to perform activities. Courts have recognized that conditions creating significant restrictions compared to the general population can qualify, even if the person can still perform the activity with effort or accommodations.

Episodic conditions like trifecta flares are specifically protected under ADA amendments. Your condition doesn't need to be consistently limiting—periods of remission don't disqualify you from coverage if the condition is substantially limiting when active.

Reasonable Accommodation Categories

Schedule modifications represent one of the most common and effective accommodations for chronic illness. This includes flexible start times, modified break schedules, part-time options, or compressed work weeks that concentrate hours into fewer days.

Work environment changes address physical limitations and environmental triggers. Examples include ergonomic furniture for EDS, air filtration systems for MCAS, temperature controls for POTS, or quiet spaces that reduce sensory overload.

Job restructuring involves modifying non-essential job functions or reassigning specific tasks that conflict with your limitations. This might include reducing standing requirements, eliminating travel, or shifting physically demanding tasks to colleagues.

Technology accommodations include assistive software for cognitive symptoms, voice recognition programs for writing difficulties, or specialized equipment that reduces physical strain during work tasks.

Leave policies encompass both scheduled medical appointments and unpredictable health needs. This includes FMLA leave, occasional sick days for flares, or extended leave for medical treatment.

The Interactive Process Framework

Accommodation requests begin a collaborative discussion between you and your employer about how to enable your success at work. This process should be ongoing and flexible as your needs change or as initial accommodations prove insufficient.

Documentation requirements vary by employer but typically include medical information confirming your condition and its functional limitations. Work with your medical team to provide clear, specific information about how your conditions affect work-related activities.

Accommodation effectiveness should be monitored and adjusted as needed. What works initially may need modification as your condition changes, job duties shift, or as you discover more effective solutions.

Employer responsibilities include good faith participation in the interactive process, implementing reasonable accommodations, and maintaining confidentiality about your medical information. Employers cannot retaliate against you for requesting accommodations.

Case Study: Successful Accommodation Implementation

Sarah, a software developer with all three trifecta conditions, worked with her employer to create a comprehensive accommodation package. Her POTS made standing meetings difficult, her MCAS reactions were triggered by strong fragrances in the office, and her EDS caused pain during long typing sessions.

The interactive process resulted in multiple accommodations: a sit-stand desk for postural flexibility, meetings scheduled in rooms without air fresheners, voice recognition software to reduce typing demands, and a modified schedule allowing her to start later when her POTS symptoms were typically better.

These accommodations cost the company less than $1,500 but enabled Sarah to maintain her productivity and advance to a senior developer position. Her success demonstrated that thoughtful accommodations often benefit both employee and employer.

Strategic Disclosure Decisions

Deciding when, how, and to whom to disclose your chronic illness requires careful consideration of your specific circumstances, workplace culture, and career goals. There's no universal right answer—the best approach depends on your individual situation.

Timing Considerations for Disclosure

Pre-employment disclosure is generally not recommended because employers cannot ask about disabilities during hiring. However, you may choose to disclose if you need accommodations during the interview process or if your condition is visible.

Post-hire disclosure timing depends on your need for accommodations, your confidence in your job performance, and your assessment of workplace culture. Some people prefer early disclosure to establish accommodations quickly, while others wait until they've proven their value.

Performance review timing can be strategic for disclosure because it occurs when your contributions are being formally recognized. However, don't wait so long that performance suffers due to lack of accommodations.

Crisis-driven disclosure often occurs when health episodes make continued silence impossible. While not ideal, crisis disclosure can still lead to positive outcomes if handled thoughtfully.

Audience Selection Strategy

Direct supervisor disclosure is often the first step because immediate managers typically handle day-to-day accommodation implementation. Choose supervisors who have shown flexibility and problem-solving skills.

Human resources involvement becomes necessary for formal accommodation requests and legal compliance. HR can also provide guidance about company policies and procedures.

Trusted colleagues may become informal supports and allies, but consider carefully who you trust with personal medical information. Start with people who have demonstrated discretion and empathy.

Team disclosure decisions depend on how your accommodations affect group dynamics and whether team members need to understand your limitations to work effectively together.

Communication Strategy Development

Condition explanation should focus on functional limitations rather than detailed medical information. Explain how your conditions affect work-related activities without providing unnecessary medical details.

Accommodation presentation frames requested modifications as solutions that enable your success rather than problems that burden the workplace. Focus on how accommodations help you contribute effectively.

Benefit demonstration shows how accommodations can improve outcomes for everyone. Flexible schedules might improve team coverage, ergonomic equipment could prevent workplace injuries, or remote work options might increase overall productivity.

Reassurance provision addresses employer concerns about costs, complexity, or precedent-setting. Provide information about accommodation effectiveness and emphasize your commitment to job performance.

Productivity Systems for Cognitive Challenges

Brain fog, fatigue, and concentration difficulties require specific strategies that help you maintain professional effectiveness despite cognitive fluctuations. These systems become particularly important in knowledge-based work that demands sustained mental effort.

Energy Management for Professional Tasks

Peak time identification helps you schedule demanding work during periods when your cognitive function is typically best. Many people with chronic illness experience better concentration in the morning, though individual patterns vary.

Task prioritization systems like the Eisenhower Matrix help you focus limited cognitive energy on high-impact activities. Categorize tasks by urgency and importance, tackling important/urgent items during peak energy periods.

Cognitive load reduction involves simplifying decision-making and routine tasks to preserve mental energy for complex work. Standardize recurring decisions, use templates for routine communications, and automate repetitive processes where possible.

Break scheduling prevents cognitive fatigue from accumulating throughout the day. Plan specific rest periods rather than working until exhaustion forces breaks. Short, frequent breaks often work better than longer, infrequent ones.

Organization and Memory Support

External memory systems compensate for brain fog and memory difficulties. Use digital calendars, task management apps, and note-taking systems to capture and organize information reliably.

Documentation habits become essential for tracking decisions, conversations, and project details that might otherwise be forgotten. Keep meeting notes, email summaries, and project logs accessible for reference.

Visual organization tools like mind maps, flowcharts, and color-coding systems can help process and retain complex information more effectively than text-heavy approaches.

Redundant systems prevent single points of failure in your organization system. Use multiple reminders for important deadlines and keep backup copies of essential information.

Technology Integration for Efficiency

Voice recognition software reduces typing demands and can be faster than keyboard input when fatigue affects manual dexterity. Modern programs have improved significantly in accuracy and ease of use.

Project management apps help track complex projects with multiple deadlines and dependencies. Choose systems that sync across devices and provide visual progress tracking.

Communication tools like video conferencing can reduce travel demands while maintaining professional relationships. Screen sharing and collaboration platforms enable effective remote participation.

Automation opportunities include email filters, calendar scheduling tools, and workflow automations that handle routine tasks without manual intervention.

Career Pivoting and Goal Adaptation

Chronic illness often requires reassessing career goals and paths, but this reassessment can lead to more satisfying and sustainable professional directions than you might have pursued otherwise.

Skills Assessment and Transferability

Core competency identification focuses on abilities that remain strong despite chronic illness. Communication skills, analytical thinking, creativity, and interpersonal abilities often persist even when physical capabilities change.

Transferable skills analysis reveals how your experience applies to different roles or industries. Project management skills from one field often transfer to others, while technical knowledge might apply in consulting or training roles.

Emerging skill development might focus on areas that align with your current capabilities and future goals. Online learning platforms make skill development accessible even with mobility or energy limitations.

Value proposition refinement helps you articulate what you bring to employers despite any limitations. Focus on unique perspectives, problem-solving abilities, and contributions that set you apart.

Alternative Career Path Exploration

Consulting opportunities allow greater schedule flexibility and the ability to choose projects that match your energy levels and interests. Many fields value experienced consultants who can work part-time or project-based.

Teaching and training roles can utilize your professional experience while often providing more flexible schedules and less physical demands than hands-on roles.

Writing and content creation leverage communication skills and can often be done on flexible schedules from home. Technical writing, particularly in healthcare or disability topics, may value your lived experience.

Hybrid roles that combine multiple interests or skills can create unique career paths that might not exist in traditional job categories but provide exactly what you need.

Remote Work Optimization

Working from home offers significant advantages for managing chronic illness, but success requires intentional setup and boundary management to maintain productivity and professional relationships.

Home Office Design for Health

Ergonomic workspace setup addresses EDS-related joint support needs with adjustable furniture, proper monitor positioning, and supportive seating that can be modified throughout the day.

Environmental control manages MCAS triggers through air filtration, temperature regulation, and control over cleaning products and fragrances used in your workspace.

Lighting optimization reduces eye strain and supports circadian rhythm regulation. Natural light when possible, supplemented with adjustable artificial lighting that can be modified based on symptoms and time of day.

Noise management creates a professional environment for video calls while providing the quiet conditions that many people with chronic illness need for concentration.

Professional Presence Maintenance

Communication protocols ensure that colleagues and supervisors stay informed about your availability and progress. Regular check-ins, status updates, and responsive communication maintain professional relationships.

Video conference optimization includes camera positioning, lighting, and background setup that presents professionally while accommodating your physical needs during meetings.

Collaboration tool mastery enables effective teamwork despite physical separation. Become proficient with platforms your team uses and suggest tools that improve accessibility for everyone.

Boundary establishment prevents remote work from becoming constant availability. Set clear work hours, create physical separation between work and rest spaces, and communicate availability expectations.

Entrepreneurship Considerations

Starting your own business offers ultimate flexibility for accommodating chronic illness, but it also requires careful planning to ensure the venture is sustainable given your health limitations.

Business Model Selection

Service-based businesses often provide more flexibility than product-based ventures because they don't require inventory management or physical production. Consulting, coaching, and professional services can often be scaled to match your energy levels.

Passive income streams through digital products, online courses, or licensing arrangements can provide revenue during health flares when active work isn't possible.

Partnership structures can distribute workload and provide backup coverage when health issues prevent your full participation. Choose partners who understand your limitations and can complement your skills.

Technology-enabled businesses leverage digital tools to minimize physical demands while maximizing reach and efficiency. Online businesses can often be managed from anywhere with internet access.

Risk Management Strategies

Financial planning for irregular income includes building larger emergency funds and diversifying revenue streams to protect against health-related work interruptions.

Health insurance considerations become critical for entrepreneurs who lose employer-provided coverage. Research marketplace options, consider spouse's coverage, or explore business insurance options.

Succession planning addresses what happens to the business during extended health absences or if your condition worsens. Document processes, train backup personnel, and consider partnerships that ensure continuity.

Professional support networks provide advice, referrals, and assistance during challenging periods. Connect with other entrepreneurs who understand both business challenges and chronic illness management.

Educational Accommodation Strategies

Students with chronic illness face unique challenges in traditional educational environments, but comprehensive accommodation plans can enable academic success while building skills for future career management.

Academic Accommodation Development

Testing modifications address cognitive symptoms and physical limitations that affect exam performance. Extended time, alternative formats, quiet testing environments, or scheduled breaks can level the playing field.

Assignment accommodations might include deadline extensions, alternative formats, or modified requirements that assess knowledge without penalizing for limitations caused by illness.

Attendance policies require careful navigation because chronic illness can create unpredictable absences. Work with disability services to establish policies that protect academic standing while accommodating medical needs.

Technology supports include access to recording devices for lectures, note-taking assistance, or software that helps manage cognitive symptoms during study sessions.

Campus Life Integration

Housing accommodations address environmental triggers, accessibility needs, and proximity to medical care. Single rooms, climate control, and reduced allergen exposure can significantly improve quality of life.

Meal plan modifications accommodate dietary restrictions for MCAS while ensuring adequate nutrition during demanding academic periods.

Transportation assistance helps navigate large campuses when mobility is limited or when POTS makes walking long distances problematic.

Emergency protocols ensure that campus health services understand your conditions and have appropriate response plans for health crises.

Workplace Culture Navigation

Building professional relationships and managing difficult colleagues requires specific strategies when chronic illness affects your work patterns or requires accommodations that others might not understand.

Ally Development Strategies

Champion identification involves finding colleagues who can advocate for inclusive policies and support your accommodation needs. Look for people in positions of influence who have shown commitment to diversity and inclusion.

Peer education helps colleagues understand chronic illness without overwhelming them with medical details. Share information about accommodations and how they help you contribute effectively.

Mentorship relationships provide career guidance from people who understand your industry while respecting your need for different approaches to professional development.

Network building focuses on quality relationships rather than quantity. Invest in connections with people who value your contributions and can provide mutual support.

Difficult Colleague Management

Resentment addressing occurs when colleagues perceive accommodations as unfair advantages. Focus on outcomes and contributions rather than process differences, and maintain professional boundaries about personal medical information.

Micromanager situations require documentation of your productivity and clear communication about how your work style achieves required results. Use objective metrics to demonstrate effectiveness.

Skeptical supervisor relationships need careful management through consistent performance, proactive communication, and gradual trust building. Focus on results and reliability within your accommodation framework.

Workplace conflict resolution uses formal channels when informal approaches fail. Document problems, involve HR when appropriate, and know your rights under disability law.

Financial Planning for Career Longevity

Chronic illness creates additional financial planning needs due to higher medical costs, potential career interruptions, and the possibility of eventual disability. Strategic planning helps build security while maintaining career flexibility.

Emergency Fund Optimization

Extended emergency funds should cover 9-12 months of expenses rather than the 3-6 months typically recommended. Higher medical costs and potential work interruptions require larger financial cushions.

Medical expense budgeting includes insurance premiums, copayments, deductibles, and out-of-pocket costs for treatments not covered by insurance. Many chronic illness patients spend 15-20% of income on medical expenses.

Income replacement planning addresses scenarios where health issues temporarily or permanently reduce earning capacity. Short-term and long-term disability insurance provide safety nets for income protection.

Healthcare cost management includes maximizing insurance benefits, using tax-advantaged accounts like HSAs, and researching patient assistance programs for expensive treatments.

Disability Insurance Considerations

Short-term disability coverage typically replaces 50-70% of income for 3-12 months and may be provided by employers or purchased individually. This coverage bridges gaps between illness onset and long-term solutions.

Long-term disability insurance becomes critical for protecting against permanent income loss. Group coverage through employers is often limited, making individual supplemental coverage advisable.

Social Security Disability Insurance provides federal benefits for qualifying disabilities but has strict requirements and long approval processes. Understanding eligibility criteria helps with planning even if you hope never to need benefits.

Return-to-work provisions in disability policies allow gradual resumption of work without immediately losing all benefits. These provisions provide flexibility for managing fluctuating conditions.

Katherine's conference room dilemma, described at the beginning of this section, resolved positively when she chose strategic disclosure. She explained her productivity patterns in terms of accommodation needs and demonstrated how her flexible schedule actually improved her output quality. Her boss, initially concerned about fairness, became an advocate when Katherine's results consistently exceeded targets despite working differently than her colleagues.

Professional success with chronic illness requires redefining achievement on your terms while building the skills and relationships that support long-term career growth. The path may look different from traditional career trajectories, but it can lead to equally meaningful and financially rewarding outcomes.

Your Professional Legacy

Career success with chronic illness often involves contributing in ways that extend beyond traditional metrics. Your problem-solving skills, resilience, and unique perspective can benefit colleagues and organizations in ways that healthy employees might not achieve.

The accommodations you advocate for and the inclusive culture you help create make workplaces better for everyone, including future employees who may face similar challenges. Your professional legacy includes not just your individual achievements but the paths you help create for others.

Moving forward, the professional skills and confidence you've developed create the foundation for the personal relationships and family dynamics covered in the next section. The advocacy skills, boundary-setting abilities, and communication strategies that serve you professionally also support healthy personal relationships.

Core Professional Development Principles

- ADA accommodation rights provide legal protection and frameworks for workplace modifications that enable professional success

- Strategic disclosure decisions require careful consideration of timing, audience, and communication strategies based on individual circumstances

- Productivity systems adapted for cognitive challenges help maintain professional effectiveness despite brain fog and fatigue fluctuations

- Career pivoting opportunities often lead to more satisfying and sustainable professional directions than original plans

- Remote work optimization addresses environmental triggers and physical limitations while maintaining professional relationships

- Entrepreneurship considerations include business model selection and risk management strategies suited to chronic illness realities

- Educational accommodations build foundation skills for lifelong career management and advocacy

- Financial planning addresses higher medical costs and potential income disruptions through emergency funds and disability insurance

Chapter 12: Relationship Dynamics

Love, Family, and Friendship with Chronic Illness

The text message from Lisa's best friend sat unanswered on her phone for three days: "You've been so distant lately. I feel like you're avoiding me." Lisa stared at the words, knowing they were true but struggling to explain that her recent MCAS flare had left her too exhausted for the chatty phone calls and impromptu dinner plans that had defined their friendship for years. How do you tell someone you love that you need them to care about you differently now? How do you maintain relationships when your energy is limited and your needs have changed?

Lisa's relationship challenge reflects one of the most painful aspects of living with chronic illness—watching important relationships strain under the weight of changed circumstances. Friends may not understand why you can't commit to plans, family members might struggle with your new limitations, and romantic partners may feel overwhelmed by the complexities of chronic illness management.

Yet many relationships actually grow stronger through the process of adapting to chronic illness. The relationships that survive often become deeper, more authentic, and more supportive than they were before illness required greater honesty and vulnerability. The key lies in learning to communicate your needs clearly, set boundaries that protect your health, and help loved ones understand how to support you effectively.

Successful relationship management with chronic illness requires both internal work—understanding your own needs and limitations—and external work—educating others about how chronic illness affects your capacity and what support looks like. This process often reveals which relationships were truly built on mutual care versus convenience or habit.

Communication Strategies for Invisible Illness

Explaining chronic illness to people who haven't experienced it requires patience, clarity, and often repeated conversations as loved ones gradually understand the realities of your condition.

The Education Framework

Basic condition explanation should focus on how illness affects daily function rather than complex medical details. "My condition affects my energy levels and makes it hard to predict how I'll feel day to day" is more useful than detailed descriptions of autonomic dysfunction.

Symptom visibility challenges require helping others understand that lack of obvious signs doesn't mean lack of real symptoms. Many people equate illness with looking sick, making invisible symptoms seem less serious or real.

Unpredictability education helps loved ones understand why you might cancel plans or seem inconsistent in your capabilities. Explain that chronic illness creates good days and bad days that can't always be predicted in advance.

Energy limitation analogies can help healthy people understand fatigue and pacing needs. The spoon theory, battery metaphors, or bank account analogies help others grasp why energy must be budgeted and conserved.

Conversation Timing and Setting

Planned discussions work better than crisis-driven explanations because they occur when you have energy to communicate clearly and loved ones can focus on understanding rather than reacting to immediate problems.

Private settings allow for honest conversation without the performance pressure of public spaces. Choose comfortable environments where both you and the other person can speak freely.

Stress-free timing avoids periods when either person is dealing with other major stressors that might interfere with understanding or empathy.

Follow-up conversations recognize that understanding chronic illness is a process, not a single conversation. Plan to revisit topics as questions arise or as your needs change.

Language and Messaging

Positive framing focuses on what you can do and what support would help rather than dwelling on limitations or complaints. "I'd love to spend time with you, and here's what would work best" is more effective than listing everything you can't do.

Specific requests provide clear guidance about how others can help rather than leaving them guessing. "Could we plan dinner for 6 PM instead of 8 PM because I have more energy earlier" is more helpful than "I'm always tired in the evenings."

Boundary communication expresses your limits kindly but firmly. "I need to leave by 9 PM to manage my symptoms" sets clear expectations while showing you value the relationship enough to participate within your limits.

Appreciation expression acknowledges when others make efforts to accommodate your needs, reinforcing positive behaviors and showing that you notice their support.

Boundary Setting for Energy Protection

Protecting your limited energy while maintaining meaningful relationships requires clear boundaries that others can understand and respect.

Energy Boundary Categories

Time boundaries include limits on visit duration, phone call length, and social event participation. These boundaries protect against overcommitment that leads to symptom flares and relationship strain.

Activity boundaries address types of activities you can and cannot participate in based on physical limitations, environmental triggers, or energy requirements. This might include avoiding crowded venues, limiting travel, or modifying traditional activities.

Emotional boundaries protect against relationships that drain more energy than they provide. This includes limiting exposure to drama, negativity, or people who consistently dismiss your health needs.

Availability boundaries communicate when you're accessible for social interaction versus when you need rest or medical care. This helps prevent hurt feelings when you can't respond immediately to calls or invitations.

Boundary Implementation Strategies

Clear communication prevents misunderstandings by stating boundaries directly rather than hoping others will guess your needs. "I can visit for two hours" is clearer than "we'll see how long I can stay."

Consistent enforcement builds respect for your boundaries while demonstrating that they're serious health needs rather than preferences you'll abandon under pressure.

Alternative suggestions show that you want to maintain the relationship within your limits. "I can't go to the concert, but could we have coffee earlier in the day?" offers connection without compromising your health.

Guilt management helps you maintain boundaries despite pressure from others who might not understand or accept your limitations. Your health needs are not negotiable, even if others disagree.

Case Study: Boundary Success

Rachel struggled with her sister's expectations for family gatherings until she implemented clear boundaries. Instead of attempting every holiday event and ending up sick, she negotiated attending one major gathering per month with specific accommodations.

Her boundaries included arrival and departure times, dietary accommodations for her MCAS, and a quiet space for breaks. Initially, family members were resistant, but Rachel's consistent participation within these boundaries eventually gained their respect and support.

The result was better relationships and better health. Rachel enjoyed family time more because she wasn't constantly managing symptoms, and family members appreciated having predictable, sustainable participation from her.

Intimacy and Physical Relationships

Chronic illness affects physical and emotional intimacy in complex ways that require open communication, creativity, and patience from both partners.

Physical Intimacy Adaptations

Energy timing coordination helps couples plan intimate moments during periods when the chronically ill partner has adequate energy and minimal symptoms. This might mean morning intimacy for people whose symptoms worsen throughout the day.

Position modifications accommodate joint hypermobility, pain, or fatigue that affect traditional approaches to physical intimacy. Open communication about what feels good and what causes problems helps couples adapt together.

Symptom management includes planning around medication timing, managing POTS symptoms through positioning, and addressing MCAS triggers that might affect intimate situations.

Pain considerations require honest communication about what's comfortable and what isn't, with flexibility to modify or postpone intimacy based on symptom levels.

Emotional Intimacy Development

Vulnerability sharing deepens relationships when partners can discuss fears, frustrations, and hopes related to chronic illness. This includes both the chronically ill partner's experiences and the healthy partner's feelings about the situation.

Support expression involves learning how to ask for and provide emotional support that feels genuine and helpful rather than overwhelming or patronizing.

Identity discussion addresses how chronic illness affects sense of self and relationship roles. Both partners may need to grieve changes in their expectations and plans.

Future planning requires honest conversation about how chronic illness might affect long-term relationship goals, family planning, and lifestyle choices.

Partner Education and Support

Medical understanding helps healthy partners learn about chronic illness symptoms, treatments, and prognosis so they can provide informed support rather than operating from fear or misunderstanding.

Advocacy skills enable partners to support their chronically ill loved ones during medical appointments, family gatherings, or social situations where advocacy might be needed.

Self-care guidance helps healthy partners maintain their own well-being while providing support. Partner burnout serves no one and actually reduces the support available to the chronically ill person.

Communication training develops skills for discussing difficult topics, managing conflicts about illness-related issues, and maintaining connection despite challenges.

Family Dynamics and Role Changes

Chronic illness often disrupts established family roles and responsibilities, requiring renegotiation of who does what and how family life operates.

Role Redistribution Strategies

Household responsibility sharing requires honest assessment of what the chronically ill family member can consistently manage versus what needs to be redistributed to others.

Financial responsibility shifts might occur if chronic illness affects earning capacity or increases medical expenses. This requires open discussion about budget changes and earning expectations.

Caregiver role definition helps family members understand what type and level of support is needed versus what constitutes overhelping that reduces independence.

Decision-making authority may need adjustment if cognitive symptoms affect the chronically ill person's ability to manage certain responsibilities consistently.

Intergenerational Considerations

Parent-child relationships require special attention when parents develop chronic illness, as children may feel scared, confused, or responsible for caregiving beyond their developmental capacity.

Adult children of chronically ill parents face decisions about how much support to provide while managing their own lives and responsibilities.

Grandparent relationships might be affected by energy limitations or activity restrictions, requiring creative approaches to maintain meaningful connections across generations.

Extended family education helps aunts, uncles, cousins, and other relatives understand chronic illness and how to maintain supportive relationships.

Family Meeting Frameworks

Regular check-ins provide opportunities to assess how role changes are working and make adjustments as needed. These don't need to be formal meetings—even brief conversations can address ongoing issues.

Problem-solving sessions address specific challenges like vacation planning, holiday traditions, or major family decisions that need to account for chronic illness limitations.

Goal-setting discussions help families plan for the future while accounting for chronic illness realities. This might include education planning, career decisions, or major purchases.

Celebration planning ensures that family achievements and milestones are recognized in ways that include everyone despite physical or energy limitations.

Dating and New Relationship Formation

Starting new romantic relationships when you have chronic illness requires deciding when and how to disclose health information while building genuine connections.

Disclosure Timing Decisions

Early disclosure allows potential partners to make informed decisions about relationship development but risks premature judgment based on limited understanding of chronic illness.

Gradual revelation involves sharing information about chronic illness progressively as emotional intimacy develops and trust builds between partners.

Activity-based disclosure might occur naturally when chronic illness affects dating activities, providing concrete examples of how conditions impact daily life.

Serious relationship disclosure becomes necessary when relationships progress toward commitment, cohabitation, or other major decisions that chronic illness might affect.

Online Dating Considerations

Profile creation decisions include choosing whether to mention chronic illness in dating profiles versus addressing it later in relationship development.

Activity planning focuses on suggesting dates that accommodate your energy levels and environmental needs while still allowing you to get to know potential partners.

Energy management prevents overcommitment during early dating when excitement might lead to ignoring your physical limitations.

Safety considerations include ensuring you have transportation options, medication access, and emergency plans during dates in unfamiliar locations.

Building Understanding with New Partners

Education pacing shares information about chronic illness gradually to avoid overwhelming new partners while ensuring they have adequate understanding for informed decision-making.

Experience sharing includes allowing new partners to observe how chronic illness affects daily life rather than just hearing descriptions of symptoms and limitations.

Support exploration helps new partners understand what types of support feel helpful versus overwhelming, and how they can contribute positively to the relationship.

Future discussion addresses how chronic illness might affect relationship goals, lifestyle choices, and major decisions that couples typically face together.

Parenting Considerations

Having and raising children with chronic illness requires careful planning and ongoing adaptation to ensure both parent and child health and well-being.

Pregnancy and Genetic Counseling

Medical consultation before conception helps assess how pregnancy might affect chronic illness symptoms and how chronic illness medications might affect fetal development.

Genetic counseling provides information about inheritance risks for conditions like EDS that have known genetic components. This information helps couples make informed decisions about family planning.

Pregnancy management requires coordination between obstetric care and chronic illness specialists to monitor both maternal health and fetal development throughout pregnancy.

Delivery planning addresses how chronic illness might affect labor and delivery options, pain management choices, and immediate postpartum care needs.

Parenting Adaptations

Energy management becomes even more critical when caring for children who depend on you for their basic needs.

This might require hiring help, accepting family support, or modifying parenting approaches.

Activity modifications help you participate in your children's lives within your physical limitations. This might include seated coaching, modified play activities, or creative alternatives to physically demanding parent-child activities.

Emergency planning ensures that children understand your health needs and know how to seek help if you experience symptoms that affect your ability to care for them.

Support network development provides backup care options for times when chronic illness symptoms prevent normal parenting activities.

Child Education About Chronic Illness

Age-appropriate explanations help children understand your health needs without creating excessive worry or responsibility for your well-being.

Routine accommodation teaches children that family life includes modifications for health needs, normalizing disability and teaching empathy and flexibility.

Emergency procedures ensure that older children know how to respond if you experience health crises, including when to call for help and who to contact.

Emotional support addresses children's feelings about having a chronically ill parent, including concerns about inheritance, family stability, and their own responsibilities.

Social Circle Management

Not all relationships will survive the changes that chronic illness brings, and learning to identify supportive versus draining relationships helps you invest your limited energy wisely.

Relationship Assessment Criteria

Energy balance evaluation considers whether specific relationships typically leave you feeling supported and energized versus drained and exhausted after interaction.

Understanding demonstration shows how well different people grasp your health needs and accommodate them versus consistently expecting you to push beyond your limits.

Consistency assessment examines whether friends and family members provide reliable support or only help when it's convenient for them.

Reciprocity analysis considers whether relationships involve mutual support and care or primarily flow in one direction, with you always giving or always receiving.

Supportive Relationship Cultivation

Investment prioritization focuses your limited social energy on relationships that provide mutual support and understanding rather than trying to maintain every previous relationship.

Appreciation expression strengthens positive relationships by acknowledging when others provide helpful support or show understanding of your health needs.

Boundary respect recognition helps you identify people who honor your limitations and support your health needs versus those who consistently push against your boundaries.

Growth opportunity identification looks for relationships that can develop deeper understanding and support through honest communication and shared experience.

Difficult Relationship Management

Minimization strategies reduce exposure to people who consistently drain your energy or dismiss your health needs while maintaining necessary family or professional relationships.

Direct communication addresses relationship problems honestly when you believe the relationship has potential for improvement through better understanding.

Professional support helps you develop skills for managing difficult relationships and deciding when to invest in relationship repair versus when to step back for your own health.

Ending relationships becomes necessary when they consistently harm your health or well-being despite efforts to improve communication and understanding.

Holiday and Event Participation

Celebrations and special events often require modifications to accommodate chronic illness while maintaining meaningful participation in important traditions and milestones.

Holiday Adaptation Strategies

Tradition modification preserves the meaning of celebrations while accommodating physical limitations and energy constraints. This might include simplified meal preparation, modified gift-giving, or altered gathering schedules.

Energy budgeting for holidays requires planning your participation in advance and building in adequate rest time before and after celebrations.

Environmental management addresses triggers like strong food odors, fragrances, temperature extremes, or crowded conditions that might worsen symptoms during celebrations.

Alternative participation options provide ways to maintain connections when traditional celebration activities aren't possible due to health limitations.

Event Planning Principles

Advance preparation reduces stress and energy expenditure during events by planning accommodations, transportation, and medication needs ahead of time.

Backup planning provides alternatives when health symptoms prevent planned participation, ensuring you don't miss important events entirely.

Communication with hosts helps event organizers understand your needs and plan accommodations that allow your participation without compromising your health.

Recovery planning includes scheduling downtime after major events to allow symptom management and energy restoration.

Lisa's text message dilemma, described at the beginning of this section, resolved when she decided to have an honest conversation with her friend about how MCAS affected her energy and availability. Instead of avoiding the relationship, she explained her limitations and suggested ways they could maintain their friendship within her health constraints. Her friend, initially hurt by the perceived distance, became one of her strongest supporters once she understood the reality of chronic illness.

Relationship management with chronic illness requires ongoing communication, patience, and willingness to help others learn how to love and support you in new ways. The relationships that adapt and grow stronger often become the most meaningful connections in your life, built on authentic understanding rather than surface-level social expectations.

The Deeper Connections Chronic Illness Creates

Living with chronic illness often filters relationships in ways that reveal their true foundation. Superficial connections based on shared activities or convenience may fade, while relationships rooted in genuine care and mutual respect often deepen. The process can be painful but ultimately creates a support network of people who see and value you as a complete person rather than just your healthy contributions.

The communication skills, boundary-setting abilities, and emotional intelligence you develop through managing relationships with chronic illness serve you throughout life. These skills often make you a better friend, partner, and family member to others facing their own challenges, creating reciprocal support systems that benefit everyone involved.

Moving forward, the relationship foundation you've built provides the support system that makes adventures, travel, and new experiences possible. Strong relationships create the safety net that allows you to take calculated risks and pursue meaningful activities despite chronic illness limitations.

Core Relationship Management Strategies

- Clear communication about invisible illness helps loved ones understand limitations and support needs without overwhelming them with medical details

- Energy-protective boundaries maintain meaningful relationships while preserving health through realistic limits on time, activities, and emotional availability

- Intimacy adaptations address physical and emotional changes while maintaining connection and mutual support between partners

- Family role redistributions acknowledge changed capabilities while maintaining family function and supporting all members' well-being

- Dating disclosure strategies balance honesty about health needs with allowing relationships to develop naturally based on compatibility and connection

- Parenting modifications ensure child safety and well-being while accommodating chronic illness limitations through planning and support systems

- Social circle assessment focuses limited energy on relationships that provide mutual support and understanding while minimizing exposure to draining dynamics

- Event participation strategies preserve meaningful traditions and celebrations through modifications that accommodate health needs without compromising connection

Chapter 13:Travel and Activity Adaptation

The travel agent's face showed polite confusion as Marcus explained his accommodation needs for the European vacation he'd been planning for two years. "So you need a hotel room near the elevator because of your joints, restaurants without strong smells because of your immune system, and activities that don't require much standing because of your heart condition?" she asked. "Are you sure you wouldn't prefer a nice staycation instead?" Marcus felt his travel dreams deflating until he remembered that the greatest adventures often require the most creative problem-solving.

Marcus's experience reflects a common assumption that chronic illness means the end of adventure, travel, and meaningful activities. Yet thousands of people with POTS, MCAS, and EDS successfully travel the world, pursue hobbies, attend concerts, and participate in outdoor activities. The difference lies not in the absence of limitations but in the presence of preparation, creativity, and adaptive strategies that make experiences accessible.

Adventure with chronic illness requires redefining what adventure means and learning to find excitement in experiences that work with your body rather than against it. Sometimes the most meaningful adventures happen close to home, while other times careful planning makes distant travel possible. The key is refusing to let perfect health be the prerequisite for a meaningful life.

Modern travel and activity industries are increasingly recognizing the needs of people with disabilities and chronic illness. Accessibility features once seen as special accommodations are now understood as universal design principles that benefit everyone. This shift creates more opportunities for people with chronic illness to participate in activities that previously seemed impossible.

Travel Planning for Complex Medical Needs

Successful travel with chronic illness starts with thorough planning that addresses medical care access, medication management, and symptom triggers while maintaining the spontaneity that makes travel enjoyable.

Destination Research Framework

Climate considerations affect all three trifecta conditions but in different ways. POTS symptoms may worsen in hot, humid climates, while MCAS reactions might increase in areas with high pollen or pollution. EDS joint pain can respond to barometric pressure changes that vary by geographic location.

Healthcare system evaluation becomes critical when traveling to areas where medical care quality or availability might differ from your home region. Research hospital locations, specialist availability, and insurance coverage for your planned destinations.

Activity accessibility assessment helps you understand what experiences will be available within your physical limitations. This includes terrain difficulty, standing requirements, environmental conditions, and availability of rest areas or accommodations.

Cultural accommodation awareness addresses how different cultures view disability and chronic illness, which can affect the support and understanding you receive while traveling.

Medical Preparation Protocols

Physician consultation before travel helps assess whether your current health status is suitable for planned activities and identifies any medication adjustments or additional preparations needed.

Medical documentation includes physician letters explaining your conditions, medication needs, and any special equipment requirements. These documents help with airport security, customs, and emergency medical care.

Medication supply management involves bringing adequate supplies for your entire trip plus extra for delays, organizing medications for easy airport security screening, and researching pharmacy availability at your destination.

Emergency contact preparation includes information for your medical team, local emergency services at your destination, and insurance company contact numbers for urgent medical needs.

Insurance and Legal Considerations

Travel insurance evaluation ensures coverage for chronic illness-related medical needs, trip cancellations due to health issues, and emergency medical evacuation if needed.

International insurance coverage requires understanding how your health insurance works abroad and whether supplemental coverage is needed for international medical care.

Prescription medication legality varies by country, and some medications available in the United States may be controlled or prohibited elsewhere. Research requirements well in advance of travel.

Emergency medical authorization documents ensure that travel companions or medical providers can make decisions on your behalf if you become unable to communicate during health emergencies.

Transportation Adaptations

Getting to destinations safely and comfortably requires understanding how different transportation methods affect chronic illness symptoms and planning accordingly.

Air Travel Optimization

Seat selection strategies include aisle seats for easy bathroom access and movement, seats near the front for quicker boarding and deplaning, and avoiding seats near galleys or lavatories that might have strong odors triggering MCAS.

Medication management during flights includes carrying all essential medications in carry-on luggage, bringing extra supplies in case of delays, and timing medication doses for time zone changes.

Hydration and circulation support becomes particularly important during long flights when POTS symptoms may worsen due to prolonged sitting and cabin pressure changes. Compression stockings, frequent movement, and electrolyte drinks help maintain circulation.

Airport accommodation requests include wheelchair assistance for long terminals, priority boarding to avoid standing in lines, and assistance with heavy luggage that might strain EDS-affected joints.

Ground Transportation Planning

Vehicle modifications for personal cars might include ergonomic seat cushions, steering wheel covers for better grip, and organizational systems for keeping medications and emergency supplies accessible.

Public transportation assessment includes understanding accessibility features, proximity to your accommodations, and backup options when primary transportation isn't suitable for your needs.

Ride-sharing considerations include communicating needs to drivers, ensuring vehicles can accommodate any mobility aids, and having backup transportation plans for situations where ride services aren't available.

Rental car accommodations involve requesting specific vehicle types that meet your needs, understanding insurance coverage for modifications, and familiarizing yourself with vehicle features before departure.

Long-Distance Travel Strategies

Pacing for multi-day journeys includes building rest days into travel itineraries, avoiding overpacked schedules that don't allow for symptom management, and planning shorter travel days when energy might be limited.

Route planning considers rest stops, medical facilities, and accommodation options along the way rather than focusing solely on reaching destinations quickly.

Emergency planning during transit includes knowing medical facility locations along your route, carrying emergency contact information, and having plans for managing health crises away from familiar medical providers.

Case Study: Successful International Travel

Sarah, who has all three trifecta conditions, successfully traveled to Europe for three weeks by implementing careful planning strategies. She researched healthcare systems in each country, obtained international health insurance, and brought a comprehensive medical kit with doctor's letters explaining her conditions.

Her preparation included booking hotels near medical facilities, researching restaurants that could accommodate her dietary restrictions, and planning a flexible itinerary that allowed for rest days when symptoms flared. She also connected with chronic illness support groups in major cities for backup emotional support.

The trip was successful because Sarah planned for her limitations rather than ignoring them. She experienced some symptom flares but had protocols in place to manage them without cutting the trip short.

Activity Modification Strategies

Adapting favorite activities and discovering new ones that work with your physical limitations opens up possibilities for meaningful experiences and continued personal growth.

Outdoor Activity Adaptations

Hiking modifications include choosing trails with appropriate difficulty levels, planning shorter distances with more rest stops, and selecting routes with good access to water and shade.

Camping accommodations might involve RV camping instead of tent camping, choosing sites with bathroom facilities, and bringing additional comfort items like supportive chairs and climate control options.

Beach and water activities require considering sun exposure that might trigger MCAS reactions, managing hydration needs in hot environments, and choosing activities that don't require prolonged standing or walking on uneven surfaces.

Nature photography and bird watching provide outdoor experiences that can be adapted for various mobility levels while still offering connection with nature and opportunities for achievement.

Cultural Activity Participation

Museum and gallery visits benefit from advance planning about accessibility features, rest areas, and crowd levels that might affect sensory sensitivity or mobility needs.

Concert and theater accommodations include accessible seating options, strategies for managing crowd noise and environmental triggers, and planning arrival and departure times to avoid peak congestion.

Festival participation requires understanding venue layouts, accessibility features, food accommodation options, and crowd management strategies that prevent overwhelming sensory experiences.

Educational workshops and classes can often be modified to accommodate chronic illness needs through seating arrangements, break schedules, and alternative participation methods.

Social Activity Adaptations

Group dining modifications include researching restaurants in advance, communicating dietary needs to hosts, and having backup food options available for situations where suitable choices aren't available.

Party and celebration strategies address energy management, environmental triggers, and exit strategies that allow participation without compromising health.

Sports event attendance includes choosing seating that accommodates mobility needs, planning for crowd noise and environmental factors, and bringing necessary supplies for comfort during long events.

Community group participation can often be modified through role adjustments, meeting accommodations, and flexible commitment levels that allow meaningful involvement without overcommitment.

Event Preparation for Special Occasions

Weddings, graduations, family reunions, and other milestone events require specific planning to ensure meaningful participation without triggering health crises.

Wedding and Celebration Planning

Venue accessibility assessment includes understanding layout, restroom locations, seating options, and environmental factors like temperature control and fragrance policies.

Dietary accommodation coordination with caterers ensures safe food options while participating in traditional celebration meals and activities.

Photography planning addresses positioning needs for joint comfort, lighting considerations for MCAS sensitivity, and timing requirements that account for energy fluctuations.

Gift and participation alternatives provide ways to contribute meaningfully to celebrations even when physical limitations affect traditional participation methods.

Family Reunion Strategies

Accommodation coordination with family members helps ensure lodging meets your accessibility and environmental needs while maintaining family connections.

Activity modification allows participation in family traditions while accommodating health limitations through role changes, timing adjustments, or alternative participation methods.

Emotional preparation addresses family dynamics that might be challenging when chronic illness affects your ability to participate in traditional ways.

Documentation planning helps capture family memories despite energy limitations through designated photographers, shared responsibility for organizing activities, and focus on quality interactions over quantity of activities.

Professional Event Participation

Conference accommodation includes requesting accessible seating, understanding venue layouts, planning rest strategies during long days, and identifying quiet spaces for managing symptoms.

Networking modifications focus on quality connections rather than quantity, strategic timing of interactions during your peak energy periods, and comfortable environments for professional conversations.

Presentation adaptations address standing requirements, microphone needs, visual presentation tools, and backup plans for managing symptoms during speaking engagements.

Follow-up strategies ensure professional connections are maintained even when health limitations affect immediate follow-through on commitments made during events.

Emergency Planning Away from Home

Managing health crises while traveling or attending events requires advance planning and clear protocols for accessing appropriate medical care in unfamiliar environments.

Medical Emergency Protocols

Local hospital identification includes researching facilities near your destination, understanding quality ratings and specialties, and knowing admission procedures and insurance requirements.

Emergency contact coordination ensures that both local emergency services and your home medical team can be reached quickly when health crises occur away from home.

Medical information accessibility includes carrying comprehensive medical summaries, current medication lists, emergency contact information, and insurance documentation in easily accessible formats.

Treatment protocol documentation helps unfamiliar medical providers understand your conditions and appropriate treatment approaches, potentially preventing harmful interventions or misdiagnosis.

Communication Strategies During Crises

Family notification systems ensure that loved ones are informed quickly about health emergencies while maintaining your privacy preferences and decision-making authority.

Medical advocacy support includes designating travel companions who can advocate for appropriate care and communicate with your regular medical team during emergencies.

Language barrier preparation for international travel includes learning key medical phrases, carrying translated medical documents, and identifying translation services available through hospitals or emergency services.

Documentation during emergencies includes keeping records of treatments received, medications administered, and follow-up instructions for coordination with your regular medical team.

Recovery Planning

Extended stay arrangements address situations where health crises require longer recovery periods before safe travel home, including accommodation modifications and care coordination.

Travel modification protocols include changing travel plans, arranging medical escorts for travel home, or modifying activities to accommodate recovery needs.

Follow-up care coordination ensures continuity between emergency treatment and your regular medical providers, including sharing medical records and treatment summaries.

Insurance claim management includes understanding coverage for emergency medical care, trip interruptions, and extended stays due to health crises.

Accommodation Strategies for Lodging

Finding suitable places to stay requires understanding accessibility features, environmental controls, and service accommodations that support your health needs.

Hotel Selection Criteria

Accessibility features assessment includes understanding room layouts, bathroom accessibility, elevator availability, and proximity to parking or transportation.

Environmental control evaluation addresses air filtration systems, cleaning product policies, fragrance-free rooms, and temperature control options that might affect MCAS symptoms.

Service accommodation policies include understanding staff training about disability needs, available assistance services, and flexibility in policies that might conflict with your health requirements.

Location considerations balance proximity to activities with access to medical facilities, pharmacies, and quiet environments that support rest and symptom management.

Alternative Accommodation Options

Vacation rental advantages include kitchen facilities for dietary management, more space for medical equipment and supplies, and greater control over environmental factors like cleaning products and air quality.

Extended stay facilities provide hotel amenities with apartment-style accommodations that might be more suitable for longer trips or when recovery time is needed.

Accessibility-focused accommodations specialize in serving people with disabilities and often provide enhanced features and staff training that support complex medical needs.

Home exchange programs can provide comfortable, familiar environments while allowing travel experiences, though they require careful coordination about accessibility and medical needs.

Preparation and Communication

Advance reservation requirements include requesting specific room features, confirming accessibility accommodations, and communicating special needs that require preparation before arrival.

Arrival coordination ensures that requested accommodations are available and that staff understand your needs for optimal service during your stay.

Room preparation includes organizing medications and medical supplies, adjusting environmental controls, and setting up communication access for emergency situations.

Service utilization includes understanding available assistance services, tipping practices for extra accommodations, and feedback systems for improving accessibility services.

Adventure Sports and Outdoor Activities

Physical limitations don't necessarily prevent participation in exciting outdoor activities, but they do require careful evaluation, preparation, and often modification of traditional approaches.

Risk Assessment Framework

Activity evaluation includes understanding physical demands, environmental risks, available safety equipment, and emergency access that might be needed during participation.

Medical clearance from your healthcare team helps ensure that planned activities are appropriate for your current health status and physical capabilities.

Guide and instructor communication ensures that activity leaders understand your limitations and can provide appropriate modifications or assistance during participation.

Emergency planning addresses how health crises would be managed during outdoor activities, including evacuation procedures and access to medical care.

Equipment and Safety Modifications

Adaptive equipment options include modifications that allow participation despite physical limitations, such as supportive seating for kayaking or stabilizing equipment for hiking.

Safety gear evaluation ensures that standard safety equipment fits properly and provides adequate protection given your specific physical needs and limitations.

Communication devices include methods for summoning help if needed, staying in contact with support teams, and coordinating with emergency services in remote locations.

Personal medical kit preparation includes medications for managing symptoms during activities, emergency supplies for health crises, and comfort items that support participation.

Modified Activity Options

Guided tour adaptations include choosing tours with appropriate pacing, accessibility features, and flexible participation options that accommodate varying energy levels.

Photography and nature observation provide outdoor experiences that can be adapted for various mobility levels while still offering meaningful engagement with natural environments.

Educational programs like nature centers, ranger programs, and outdoor workshops often provide outdoor experiences with built-in accommodations and flexible participation options.

Volunteer opportunities in outdoor settings can provide meaningful engagement with nature and conservation while accommodating physical limitations through role modifications.

Marcus's European adventure, described at the beginning of this section, became one of his most memorable experiences after he found a travel agent who specialized in accessible travel. Together, they designed an itinerary that included adapted city tours, accessible accommodations, and carefully planned rest periods that allowed him to experience European culture within his physical limitations.

Adventure with chronic illness often requires more creativity and planning than traditional travel, but it can also lead to more meaningful experiences and greater appreciation for the opportunities that careful preparation makes possible. The problem-solving skills you develop in adapting activities often lead to innovations that benefit other travelers with similar needs.

Expanding Your Definition of Adventure

Living with chronic illness often expands your definition of what constitutes adventure and meaningful experience. A successful day trip might represent as much achievement and enjoyment as an international vacation once did. This shift in perspective often leads to greater appreciation for accessible experiences and deeper satisfaction from accomplishments that work within your limitations.

The planning skills, advocacy abilities, and adaptability you develop through accessible travel serve you well beyond vacation planning. These skills transfer to managing daily life challenges, workplace accommodations, and social activities that require similar problem-solving approaches.

Moving forward, the confidence and experience you've gained through accessible adventures provide the foundation for addressing the mental health aspects of chronic illness covered in the next section. Success in adapting meaningful activities often supports psychological well-being and identity development beyond illness.

Essential Adventure Accessibility Principles

- Thorough travel planning addresses medical needs, destination research, and emergency protocols while maintaining flexibility for spontaneous experiences

- Transportation adaptations ensure safe, comfortable transit through strategic planning for air travel, ground transportation, and long-distance journeys

- Activity modifications preserve meaningful experiences through creative adaptations that work with physical limitations rather than against them

- Event preparation strategies enable participation in special occasions through advance planning, accommodation coordination, and flexible participation approaches

- Emergency planning protocols provide safety nets for managing health crises away from familiar medical providers and support systems

- Accommodation strategies address lodging needs through accessibility assessment, environmental control, and service coordination that support health requirements

- Adventure sports adaptations allow participation in exciting outdoor activities through risk assessment, equipment modification, and safety planning that accommodate chronic illness limitations

Chapter 14: Mental Health Integration

Psychological Wellness in Chronic Illness

The therapist's office felt strangely foreign to Dr. Jennifer Walsh, despite her own training in psychology. Six months after her POTS diagnosis, she found herself on the other side of the therapeutic relationship, struggling to articulate the grief she felt for her pre-illness identity. "I used to be the person who never got sick, who powered through everything," she told her therapist. "Now I need naps and can't stand for long periods. I know intellectually that I'm still valuable, but I feel like I've lost myself." Her training had prepared her to help others navigate mental health challenges, but nothing had prepared her for the psychological complexity of chronic illness.

Jennifer's experience reflects the reality that chronic illness affects far more than physical health—it fundamentally challenges your sense of self, your future plans, and your understanding of what life should look like. The psychological impact often receives less attention than symptom management, yet mental health significantly affects physical symptoms, treatment adherence, and overall quality of life.

The relationship between mental and physical health becomes particularly complex in trifecta conditions where stress can trigger symptom flares, depression can worsen fatigue, and anxiety can intensify POTS symptoms. This interconnection means that addressing psychological wellness isn't separate from managing physical health—it's an essential component of overall treatment.

Mental health support for chronic illness requires understanding that psychological responses to real physical limitations are different from primary mental health conditions. Grief about lost abilities is normal. Anxiety about unpredictable symptoms is rational. Depression in response to life changes is understandable. The goal isn't to eliminate these responses but to process them healthily while building coping skills that support long-term well-being.

Grief and Loss Processing

Chronic illness involves multiple losses that require active grieving to process healthily. These losses often go unrecognized by others, making the grieving process particularly challenging and isolating.

Types of Losses in Chronic Illness

Physical capability losses include activities you can no longer perform safely or enjoyably due to symptoms or physical limitations. This might include sports, dancing, hiking, or work tasks that once brought satisfaction and identity.

Identity losses affect your sense of who you are when illness changes your capabilities, roles, or self-perception. The person who prided themselves on reliability might struggle when illness makes commitments unpredictable.

Future plan disruptions include career goals, travel plans, family planning decisions, or retirement dreams that need modification due to chronic illness realities.

Relationship changes involve losses when some friendships can't adapt to chronic illness needs, when family dynamics shift due to caregiving roles, or when social activities become inaccessible.

Independence reductions affect your ability to manage daily life without assistance, accommodation, or modification. This includes everything from driving limitations to needing help with household tasks.

The Grief Process in Chronic Illness

Denial often appears as minimizing symptoms, pushing through limitations without accommodations, or believing that perfect treatment adherence will restore full health.

Anger may be directed toward medical providers who can't cure your conditions, family members who don't understand your limitations, or toward your own body for its perceived betrayal.

Bargaining involves attempts to negotiate with your illness—promising perfect diet adherence, supplement regimens, or lifestyle changes in exchange for symptom relief.

Depression reflects the sadness and hopelessness that can accompany realization that some losses may be permanent and that life will be different than originally planned.

Acceptance doesn't mean being happy about chronic illness but rather acknowledging reality and working within it to build a meaningful life despite limitations.

Complicated Grief Recognition

Prolonged grief becomes concerning when normal grieving processes become stuck, preventing adaptation and forward movement for extended periods.

Disenfranchised grief occurs when losses aren't recognized or validated by others, making the grieving process more difficult and isolating.

Ambiguous loss characterizes the experience of living with chronic illness where you're neither fully healthy nor completely disabled, creating uncertainty about what to grieve and what to hope for.

Anticipatory grief involves mourning future losses that haven't occurred yet but seem likely, such as disease progression or worsening limitations.

Anxiety Management for Health-Related Fears

Anxiety about health symptoms, medical appointments, and future disease progression is common and often rational, but it can become overwhelming and interfere with daily functioning when not managed effectively.

Types of Health Anxiety

Symptom monitoring anxiety involves excessive focus on bodily sensations and fear that normal fluctuations indicate serious problems or disease progression.

Medical appointment anxiety includes fear of receiving bad news, concern about being believed by medical providers, or worry about advocating effectively for your needs.

Treatment anxiety encompasses fears about medication side effects, invasive procedures, or the possibility that treatments won't be effective.

Future progression anxiety involves worry about how chronic illness might worsen over time and affect your ability to maintain current lifestyle and relationships.

Social anxiety related to chronic illness includes fear of symptom episodes in public, concern about others' reactions to your limitations, or worry about being judged for your accommodations.

Anxiety Management Strategies

Cognitive restructuring helps identify and challenge anxious thoughts that may be exaggerated or unrealistic while acknowledging legitimate concerns that require attention.

Exposure therapy gradually increases tolerance for anxiety-provoking situations like medical appointments or social activities, building confidence and reducing avoidance behaviors.

Relaxation techniques including deep breathing, progressive muscle relaxation, and mindfulness meditation can help manage both anxiety symptoms and chronic illness symptoms that anxiety might worsen.

Practical preparation reduces anxiety through concrete planning for challenging situations, such as preparing questions for medical appointments or planning accommodations for social events.

Medical PTSD Recognition

Medical trauma can result from frightening medical experiences, dismissive medical providers, painful procedures, or life-threatening health episodes that create lasting psychological impact.

Symptoms of medical PTSD include flashbacks to traumatic medical experiences, avoidance of medical care even when needed, hypervigilance about symptoms, and emotional numbing related to health issues.

Recovery approaches include trauma-focused therapy, gradual re-exposure to medical settings with support, and building trusting relationships with new medical providers who understand trauma responses.

Depression Recognition and Management

Depression in chronic illness can be both a response to illness-related losses and a separate condition that requires specific treatment. Understanding the difference helps guide appropriate intervention approaches.

Distinguishing Situational from Clinical Depression

Situational depression represents normal emotional responses to chronic illness challenges, including sadness about limitations, frustration with symptoms, and discouragement about treatment difficulties.

Clinical depression involves persistent symptoms that significantly impair functioning beyond what would be expected from illness-related challenges alone.

Symptom overlap between depression and chronic illness includes fatigue, sleep disturbances, concentration difficulties, and reduced interest in activities, making diagnosis challenging.

Duration and severity considerations help distinguish between normal adjustment reactions and depression requiring clinical intervention.

Depression Treatment Approaches

Therapy modalities effective for chronic illness-related depression include cognitive-behavioral therapy, acceptance and commitment therapy, and chronic illness-specific counseling approaches.

Medication considerations require understanding how antidepressants might interact with chronic illness treatments and how they might affect symptoms of conditions like POTS or MCAS.

Lifestyle interventions including regular exercise within physical limitations, social connection maintenance, and meaningful activity engagement can help manage both depression and chronic illness symptoms.

Support group participation provides connection with others facing similar challenges and reduces the isolation that often contributes to depression in chronic illness.

Suicidal Ideation in Chronic Illness

Risk factors for suicidal thoughts in chronic illness include inadequate pain management, social isolation, financial stress from medical costs, and hopelessness about future quality of life.

Warning signs include talking about feeling hopeless, making statements about being a burden to others, withdrawing from relationships, or making preparations that suggest planning for death.

Intervention approaches include immediate safety planning, increasing support and supervision, addressing treatable factors like pain or depression, and connecting with mental health crisis services.

Prevention strategies focus on building strong support networks, maintaining hope through goal-setting and meaningful activities, and ensuring adequate treatment for both physical and mental health symptoms.

Building Resilience and Coping Skills

Resilience in chronic illness involves developing the psychological flexibility to adapt to changing circumstances while maintaining a sense of purpose and well-being despite ongoing challenges.

Resilience Components

Adaptability involves developing flexibility in goals, expectations, and approaches to challenges rather than rigidly adhering to pre-illness plans and methods.

Meaning-making helps find purpose and significance in experiences, including chronic illness, rather than viewing illness only as a loss or failure.

Self-efficacy includes maintaining confidence in your ability to manage challenges and influence outcomes despite the limitations chronic illness might impose.

Social connection provides emotional support, practical assistance, and sense of belonging that buffers against stress and promotes resilience.

Coping Strategy Development

Problem-focused coping addresses challenges that can be changed through action, such as finding better medical providers, implementing accommodations, or modifying activities.

Emotion-focused coping helps manage feelings and stress responses to challenges that can't be changed, such as grieving losses or accepting permanent limitations.

Meaning-focused coping involves finding positive significance in difficult experiences, such as personal growth, increased empathy, or deeper relationships that result from chronic illness challenges.

Avoidance coping includes healthy temporary disengagement from overwhelming stressors as well as problematic long-term avoidance that prevents adaptation and problem-solving.

Post-Traumatic Growth

Personal strength recognition involves acknowledging the resilience and capabilities you've developed through managing chronic illness challenges.

Relationship deepening often occurs as chronic illness reveals which relationships provide genuine support and leads to more authentic, meaningful connections with others.

Life appreciation may increase as chronic illness creates greater awareness of health, relationships, and experiences that were previously taken for granted.

Spiritual development can involve strengthened religious faith, increased sense of connection to others and the world, or development of personal philosophy that provides meaning and guidance.

Therapy Modalities for Chronic Illness

Different therapeutic approaches offer various benefits for addressing the psychological aspects of chronic illness, and finding the right fit requires understanding what each modality offers.

Cognitive Behavioral Therapy Adaptations

CBT for chronic illness focuses on identifying and changing thought patterns and behaviors that worsen symptoms or interfere with adaptation to illness.

Thought challenging techniques help distinguish between realistic concerns about chronic illness and catastrophic thinking that increases distress without improving outcomes.

Behavioral activation addresses depression and isolation by gradually increasing meaningful activities and social connections within physical limitations.

Pacing and energy management strategies help balance activity and rest to prevent symptom flares while maintaining engagement in valued activities.

Acceptance and Commitment Therapy

Psychological flexibility development helps you respond to chronic illness challenges based on your values rather than being controlled by difficult thoughts and emotions.

Values clarification identifies what matters most to you and guides decision-making about how to live meaningfully despite chronic illness limitations.

Mindfulness skills help you observe thoughts and feelings about chronic illness without being overwhelmed by them or needing to eliminate them completely.

Committed action involves taking steps toward valued goals even when chronic illness creates obstacles or uncertainty about outcomes.

Trauma-Informed Approaches

Medical trauma processing addresses specific traumatic experiences in healthcare settings that may affect current medical care engagement and emotional well-being.

Body awareness restoration helps rebuild trust and connection with your body after chronic illness may have created fear or disconnection from physical sensations.

Safety and control rebuilding focuses on regaining sense of agency and empowerment in medical care and daily life after traumatic health experiences.

Group Therapy Benefits

Peer support provides connection with others who understand chronic illness challenges firsthand, reducing isolation and normalizing difficult experiences.

Skill sharing allows group members to learn from each other's coping strategies and practical solutions for chronic illness management.

Mutual aid creates opportunities to help others facing similar challenges, which often provides sense of purpose and increased self-efficacy.

Accountability support helps maintain motivation for therapy goals and healthy behaviors through gentle peer encouragement and check-ins.

Medication Considerations for Mental Health

Psychiatric medications in chronic illness require careful consideration of interactions with other treatments and effects on chronic illness symptoms.

Antidepressant Selection

SSRI considerations include understanding how these medications might affect POTS symptoms, interact with other medications, or influence conditions like MCAS.

Tricyclic antidepressants may be used for both depression and chronic pain management but require monitoring for cardiovascular effects in POTS patients.

Atypical antidepressants like bupropion may be preferred when traditional antidepressants cause problematic side effects or don't address specific symptom combinations.

Anti-Anxiety Medications

Benzodiazepine use requires careful consideration because these medications can affect blood pressure and heart rate regulation in POTS patients.

Buspirone and other non-benzodiazepine anti-anxiety medications may be preferred for long-term anxiety management in chronic illness.

Medication Timing and Interactions

Dose timing affects both psychiatric symptoms and chronic illness symptoms, requiring coordination between mental health providers and other medical specialists.

Interaction monitoring becomes particularly important when psychiatric medications are added to complex chronic illness treatment regimens.

Case Study: Integrated Mental Health Treatment

Maria developed significant depression and anxiety following her trifecta diagnosis, which worsened her physical symptoms and interfered with her ability to manage her medical care effectively.

Her treatment team included a psychiatrist familiar with chronic illness who prescribed an SSRI that didn't worsen her POTS symptoms, a therapist specializing in chronic illness who provided CBT and acceptance-based interventions, and coordination with her medical team to ensure integrated care.

The combination of medication and therapy helped Maria develop coping skills for managing symptom unpredictability, process grief about her changed life plans, and build confidence in advocating for her medical needs. Her mental health improvement also led to better physical symptom management and improved quality of life.

Identity Reconstruction Beyond Illness

Chronic illness often requires rebuilding your sense of self to include illness management while maintaining other important aspects of identity and purpose.

Identity Integration Strategies

Whole person recognition involves acknowledging that you are more than your chronic illness while also accepting that illness management is part of your current reality.

Strength identification focuses on capabilities, qualities, and achievements that persist despite chronic illness rather than only focusing on limitations and losses.

Role adaptation involves modifying how you fulfill important roles like parent, partner, employee, or friend rather than abandoning these roles entirely.

New identity development may include discovering interests, capabilities, or purposes that emerge through chronic illness experiences.

Value-Based Living

Personal values clarification helps identify what matters most to you independent of health status, providing guidance for decision-making and goal-setting.

Goal modification adapts aspirations to current realities while maintaining meaningful pursuits that align with your core values.

Legacy consideration involves thinking about how you want to contribute to others and the world despite or because of your chronic illness experience.

Meaning-Making Processes

Narrative therapy techniques help you rewrite your life story to include chronic illness as one chapter rather than the entire story.

Benefit finding involves identifying positive changes or growth that have resulted from chronic illness challenges without minimizing the real difficulties involved.

Purpose development may include using your chronic illness experience to help others, advocate for change, or pursue goals that have become more important due to illness.

Jennifer's therapeutic journey, described at the beginning of this section, led her to a deeper understanding of both her professional work and her personal experience with chronic illness. Her therapy helped her process the grief of lost identity while discovering new aspects of herself that emerged through managing chronic illness. She eventually specialized in working with healthcare professionals who develop chronic illness, using her dual perspective to provide uniquely informed support.

Mental health integration in chronic illness requires understanding that psychological responses to real physical challenges are different from primary mental health conditions. The goal isn't to achieve perfect mental health despite chronic illness but to develop the coping skills, support systems, and sense of purpose that enable psychological well-being alongside ongoing health challenges.

Psychological Wellness as Foundation

Mental health provides the foundation that supports all other aspects of chronic illness management. When psychological well-being is stable, you're better able to advocate for medical care, maintain relationships, pursue meaningful activities, and adapt to the ongoing challenges that chronic illness presents.

The coping skills, self-awareness, and resilience you develop through addressing mental health aspects of chronic illness serve you throughout life and often enable you to support others facing similar challenges.

Moving forward, the psychological stability and self-awareness you've developed create the foundation for building the community connections and support systems covered in the next section. Strong mental health enables you to both seek and provide support in ways that benefit both you and others.

Core Mental Health Integration Elements

- Grief processing acknowledges multiple losses from chronic illness while supporting healthy adaptation and acceptance of changed circumstances

- Anxiety management addresses rational health fears while preventing excessive worry from interfering with daily functioning and medical care engagement

- Depression recognition distinguishes between normal adjustment reactions and clinical depression requiring specific intervention approaches

- Resilience building develops psychological flexibility and coping skills that support adaptation to ongoing chronic illness challenges

- Therapy modalities provide specialized approaches for addressing chronic illness-specific mental health needs through trained professionals

- Medication considerations balance psychiatric treatment needs with chronic illness symptoms and medication interactions

- Identity reconstruction integrates chronic illness experience into a broader sense of self that includes but isn't defined by health conditions

Chapter 15:Creating Your Support Ecosystem

The notification chimed on Dr. Amanda Chen's phone at 2 AM as she lay awake with another MCAS flare. Instead of feeling isolated in her symptoms, she opened her chronic illness support group chat to find three other members also awake and struggling. "Anyone else having a rough night?" she typed, and within minutes received responses offering practical advice, emotional support, and the simple comfort of knowing she wasn't alone. What had started as an online search for POTS information two years earlier had evolved into a network of relationships that provided more understanding and practical support than many of her long-term friendships.

Amanda's experience illustrates the transformative power of community in chronic illness management. While family and friends provide essential support, they often can't fully understand the daily realities of living with complex medical conditions. Fellow patients offer a different type of support—practical advice from lived experience, validation of struggles that seem invisible to others, and hope from seeing others thrive despite similar challenges.

Building community with chronic illness requires intention and strategy because traditional social structures often don't accommodate the realities of fluctuating symptoms, energy limitations, and medical needs. You need to actively seek out connections with people who understand your experience while also contributing to communities in ways that match your capabilities and energy levels.

Modern technology has revolutionized community building for people with chronic illness, creating opportunities for connection that transcend geographic limitations and schedule constraints. Yet these same tools require careful navigation to avoid information overload, comparison traps, and the emotional exhaustion that can come from constant exposure to others' medical struggles.

Online Communities and Digital Connections

Digital platforms provide unprecedented access to people sharing similar health experiences, but success requires understanding how to navigate these spaces safely and productively.

Platform Selection and Evaluation

Facebook groups offer large, active communities with diverse membership but may lack moderation quality and include commercial promotion that interferes with genuine support.

Reddit communities provide anonymous discussion spaces with good moderation systems but may include harsh criticism or overwhelming technical information that increases anxiety.

Discord servers create real-time chat opportunities with smaller, more intimate groups but require more active engagement and may feel overwhelming for people with limited energy.

Specialized platforms like PatientsLikeMe or condition-specific websites offer focused communities with structured information sharing but may have smaller user bases.

Safe Participation Guidelines

Privacy protection includes using usernames that don't reveal personal information, being cautious about sharing location details, and understanding platform privacy settings.

Information verification involves fact-checking medical advice with qualified healthcare providers rather than relying solely on peer experiences for treatment decisions.

Emotional boundaries help protect against taking on others' distress, avoiding comparison traps that worsen mood, and limiting exposure when community participation becomes draining.

Constructive engagement focuses on offering support based on your experience while avoiding giving specific medical advice or making claims about treatments you haven't personally tried.

Digital Wellness Strategies

Time limits prevent online community participation from consuming excessive energy or replacing offline relationships and activities.

Notification management reduces the constant stimulation that can worsen symptoms while ensuring you don't miss important support when needed.

Content curation involves following accounts and joining groups that provide helpful information and support while unfollowing sources that increase anxiety or distress.

Break periods include planned time away from online communities to prevent burnout and maintain perspective on your own health journey separate from others' experiences.

Local Support Group Development

In-person connections provide different benefits than online communities, including practical assistance, local resource sharing, and the comfort of face-to-face interaction.

Finding Existing Groups

Hospital and clinic networks often sponsor support groups for specific conditions or general chronic illness experiences. Contact social workers or patient advocates at medical facilities for information.

Community centers, libraries, and religious organizations may host health-related support groups or have space available for starting new groups.

Patient advocacy organizations frequently maintain directories of local support groups and can provide information about starting new groups in underserved areas.

Meetup platforms and similar services help identify informal gatherings of people with shared health experiences in your geographic area.

Starting Your Own Group

Needs assessment involves determining what type of support group would be most helpful in your area, considering factors like condition focus, age ranges, and meeting formats.

Location identification includes finding accessible, affordable meeting spaces that accommodate mobility needs and provide comfortable environments for sharing personal information.

Structure development involves deciding on meeting frequency, format, and leadership approaches that create supportive environments without becoming overwhelming for organizers.

Promotion strategies help attract members through medical provider referrals, community bulletin boards, and online platforms while maintaining privacy and safety.

Group Facilitation Skills

Active listening techniques help create safe spaces where members feel heard and validated without requiring professional counseling training.

Boundary setting includes establishing group guidelines about confidentiality, giving advice, and maintaining focus on support rather than medical information sharing.

Conflict resolution skills help address disagreements or personality conflicts that might arise in group settings without damaging the supportive environment.

Inclusion practices ensure that group dynamics welcome people with varying symptom severities, backgrounds, and support needs.

Advocacy Opportunities and Giving Back

Contributing to chronic illness communities provides purpose and meaning while creating positive change for others facing similar challenges.

Individual Advocacy Approaches

Healthcare provider education involves sharing resources about chronic illness with medical providers who may lack knowledge about conditions like POTS, MCAS, or EDS.

Workplace accommodation advocacy includes modeling successful accommodation requests and sharing information with human resources departments about disability rights and chronic illness needs.

Family and friend education helps expand understanding and support in your immediate circle while potentially benefiting others in their networks who develop chronic illness.

Social media awareness campaigns can increase visibility of chronic illness experiences and reduce stigma through authentic sharing of your story and experiences.

Organizational Involvement

Patient advocacy organizations like Dysautonomia International, The Mastocytosis Society, and The Ehlers-Danlos Society offer volunteer opportunities that match various energy levels and skill sets.

Research participation includes joining patient registries, participating in surveys, and contributing to studies that advance understanding of chronic illness.

Fundraising activities support research and patient services through events and campaigns that can be adapted for different participation levels and physical capabilities.

Policy advocacy involves contacting legislators about healthcare access, disability rights, and research funding issues that affect chronic illness communities.

Mentorship and Peer Support

Newly diagnosed support includes sharing practical advice and emotional support with people beginning their chronic illness journey.

Skill sharing involves teaching others about topics like medical advocacy, workplace accommodations, or daily management strategies you've successfully developed.

Hope modeling demonstrates that meaningful life is possible with chronic illness through your example of adaptation and achievement despite health challenges.

Experience documentation through blogs, videos, or other formats helps preserve and share knowledge that benefits others facing similar situations.

Professional Networking in Chronic Illness Spaces

Building career connections within chronic illness communities creates opportunities for professional development while working with people who understand your health needs.

Industry-Specific Networks

Healthcare professional groups for practitioners with chronic illness provide career support and opportunities to improve care for others with similar conditions.

Technology sector networks connect people using skills in accessibility, health tech development, or digital health solutions that benefit chronic illness communities.

Legal professional associations focus on disability rights, healthcare law, or workplace accommodation issues that affect people with chronic illness.

Creative industry groups support artists, writers, and content creators who address chronic illness themes or work within health limitations.

Entrepreneurship Communities

Chronic illness entrepreneur networks provide business support specifically for people building companies while managing health challenges.

Social enterprise development focuses on businesses that address chronic illness needs while providing sustainable employment for people with health limitations.

Consulting and freelance networks offer flexible work opportunities that accommodate unpredictable symptoms and medical appointments.

Skill Development and Training

Accessible education programs provide professional development opportunities designed for people with chronic illness and disability.

Mentorship matching connects experienced professionals with chronic illness to newcomers seeking career guidance.

Conference accessibility advocacy works to improve professional event accessibility while creating networking opportunities within chronic illness communities.

Family Support Systems and Education

Helping family members understand and support your chronic illness journey requires ongoing education and communication while respecting their own emotional needs.

Immediate Family Integration

Spouse and partner support includes education about chronic illness realities, communication about changing needs, and strategies for maintaining relationship intimacy despite health challenges.

Parent education for adult children with chronic illness involves helping parents understand their adult child's autonomy while providing appropriate support and advocacy.

Sibling dynamics may require addressing feelings of guilt, responsibility, or resentment that can arise when chronic illness affects family relationships and responsibilities.

Children's understanding when parents have chronic illness includes age-appropriate education about health conditions and ensuring children don't feel responsible for caregiving beyond their developmental capacity.

Extended Family Engagement

Holiday and gathering modifications help extended family understand accommodation needs while preserving meaningful traditions and connections.

Communication strategies address questions and concerns from relatives who may not understand chronic illness or may hold outdated beliefs about disability and health.

Advocacy training helps family members support you effectively in medical, social, and workplace situations where additional voices might be helpful.

Boundary establishment protects both your health needs and family relationships by setting clear expectations about support, visits, and participation in family activities.

Educational Resources and Tools

Condition-specific materials from patient advocacy organizations provide reliable information that family members can review independently.

Video resources and documentaries help family members understand chronic illness experiences through visual and narrative formats that may be more engaging than written materials.

Family therapy or counseling provides professional support for addressing chronic illness impacts on family dynamics and relationships.

Support groups for family members of people with chronic illness offer education and emotional support from others in similar situations.

Crisis Support Networks

Building emergency emotional support systems ensures that help is available during acute mental health crises or overwhelming symptom flares.

Emergency Contact Systems

Tiered support networks include primary contacts for immediate crisis support, secondary contacts for ongoing support needs, and professional crisis services for emergency situations.

Communication protocols establish how and when to contact different support people, including preferences for phone calls, texts, or in-person assistance.

Geographic considerations ensure that both local and remote support options are available depending on the type of crisis and support needed.

Professional integration includes mental health crisis services, medical emergency contacts, and coordination between peer support and professional care.

Proactive Crisis Planning

Warning sign recognition helps both you and your support network identify early signs of developing mental health crises or overwhelming symptom periods.

Intervention strategies provide specific actions that support people can take to help during different types of crises, from practical assistance to emotional support.

Professional trigger protocols establish when peer support should transition to professional mental health or medical intervention.

Recovery support includes assistance during the period following crises when you may need ongoing help but may not be in immediate danger.

Mutual Aid and Reciprocal Support

Peer support exchange creates relationships where support flows in multiple directions rather than one person always giving or receiving help.

Skill and resource sharing allows community members to contribute different types of support based on their capabilities and circumstances.

Collective advocacy amplifies individual voices through group action on issues affecting the chronic illness community.

Community resilience building strengthens the entire support network's ability to help members during difficult periods.

Volunteer Opportunities Within Physical Limitations

Contributing to causes you care about provides purpose and connection while working within your energy and physical constraints.

Adapted Volunteer Roles

Administrative support includes tasks like data entry, phone calls, or correspondence that can often be done from home on flexible schedules.

Social media and communication roles leverage digital skills to help organizations reach audiences and share information about their missions.

Peer support positions utilize your lived experience with chronic illness to help others while providing training and support for the volunteer role.

Research and writing projects contribute to knowledge development and resource creation for chronic illness communities.

Flexible Commitment Options

Project-based volunteering allows contribution to specific initiatives without ongoing time commitments that might become difficult to maintain.

Seasonal opportunities provide ways to help during specific times of year when your health might be more stable or when organizations have particular needs.

Remote participation enables volunteering from home, reducing travel demands and environmental triggers while still providing meaningful contribution.

Team approaches distribute responsibilities among multiple volunteers, reducing individual pressure while maintaining collective impact.

Organization Selection Criteria

Mission alignment ensures that your volunteer efforts support causes you genuinely care about, providing motivation during difficult health periods.

Accessibility awareness indicates organizations that understand and accommodate volunteers with disabilities and chronic illness.

Flexibility policies demonstrate organizational commitment to adapting volunteer roles to individual capabilities and changing needs.

Support provision includes training, supervision, and assistance that helps volunteers succeed while managing chronic illness challenges.

Amanda's 2 AM support group interaction, described at the beginning of this section, represents one moment in a community network that has provided her with practical advice, emotional support, research opportunities, and meaningful ways to help others. Her online connections led to local meetups, volunteer opportunities, and professional networking that enriched her life far beyond medical support.

Community building with chronic illness creates networks that often become more supportive and understanding than traditional social structures. These communities provide practical assistance, emotional validation, advocacy opportunities, and the sense of purpose that comes from helping others navigate similar challenges.

The Ripple Effects of Community Connection

The support you receive from chronic illness communities often motivates you to provide support to others, creating positive cycles that strengthen the entire network. Your questions help others think through similar decisions, your successes provide hope during difficult times, and your challenges remind others that they're not alone in their struggles.

Community involvement often leads to personal growth and skill development that extends beyond health management. Advocacy skills improve professional abilities, peer support develops emotional intelligence, and leadership opportunities build confidence that transfers to other life areas.

The communities you build and contribute to become part of your legacy, creating support systems that will help future people diagnosed with chronic illness while honoring the challenges you've faced and overcome.

Core Community Building Principles

- Online community participation requires platform selection, safety guidelines, and digital wellness strategies that maximize benefits while minimizing risks

- Local support group development creates in-person connections through finding existing groups or starting new ones that meet specific community needs

- Advocacy opportunities provide meaningful ways to contribute to positive change while working within physical and energy limitations

- Professional networking within chronic illness spaces creates career opportunities with people who understand health accommodation needs

- Family support system education helps loved ones provide effective assistance while maintaining healthy relationship boundaries

- Crisis support networks ensure emergency emotional and practical assistance during acute mental health or symptom crises

- Volunteer opportunities adapted for chronic illness provide purpose and community contribution within realistic physical and energy constraints

Quick Reference Guides

Emergency Contact Templates

Medical Information Card Format

Your emergency medical information card should fit in your wallet and include essential details that first responders and emergency medical staff need immediately. The front of the card should contain your name, date of birth, emergency contacts, and primary medical conditions. List "POTS (Postural Orthostatic Tachycardia Syndrome), MCAS (Mast Cell Activation Syndrome), EDS (Ehlers-Danlos Syndrome)" clearly at the top.

Include your primary care physician's name and phone number, along with your most important specialist contacts. Emergency contacts should include at least two people who understand your medical conditions and can advocate for you if you're unable to communicate effectively.

The back of the card should list current medications with dosages, known drug allergies, and any critical medical alerts. For trifecta patients, important alerts might include "Prone to fainting - requires slow position changes," "Multiple environmental allergies," or "Joint hypermobility - handle carefully."

Digital Emergency Information

Create digital copies of your emergency information using your phone's emergency contact features and medical ID functions. Both iPhone and Android devices allow you to store medical information that's accessible even when your phone is locked.

Include the same information as your physical card but with room for more detail. Add information about your preferred hospital, insurance details, and specific instructions like "Contact Dr. [Name] at [Clinic] for POTS management" or "Carries EpiPen for severe allergic reactions."

Store backup copies in cloud services like Google Drive or Dropbox, ensuring family members know how to access this information during emergencies. Share your emergency information with trusted family members and update it whenever medications or contact information changes.

Travel Emergency Cards

When traveling, create modified emergency cards that include information relevant to your destination. Add embassy contact information for international travel, travel insurance details, and local emergency service numbers.

Include your home medical team's contact information along with any local medical contacts you've researched before traveling. Note any language barriers and include translated phrases for key medical terms in the local language.

Medication Lists

Comprehensive Medication Tracking Template

Your medication list should include prescription medications, over-the-counter drugs, supplements, and any herbal remedies you use regularly. For each medication, record the generic name, brand name, dosage, frequency, prescribing physician, and the condition it treats.

Include the pharmacy information where each prescription is filled, as this helps during emergencies or when traveling.

Note any specific timing requirements, such as "Take with food" or "Take 2 hours before other medications."

Track start dates for new medications and note any dose changes with dates. This information helps identify patterns between medication changes and symptom improvements or side effects.

Side Effect and Effectiveness Tracking

Create a section for documenting how well each medication works and any side effects you experience. Use a simple scale (1-10) to rate effectiveness and note any patterns related to timing, food intake, or other factors.

Document any medications you've tried in the past that didn't work well, including the reasons for discontinuation. This prevents repetitive trials of ineffective treatments and helps new medical providers understand your treatment history.

Include emergency medications and when to use them. For MCAS patients, this might include "Take additional Benadryl if experiencing flushing and rapid heart rate" or "Use EpiPen if experiencing difficulty breathing or severe whole-body reaction."

Insurance and Cost Information

Track insurance coverage for each medication, including copay amounts and any prior authorization requirements. Note which medications require specialty pharmacy ordering or have specific insurance restrictions.

Document any patient assistance programs you use and their renewal dates. Include contact information for pharmaceutical company patient assistance programs and eligibility requirements.

Symptom Diaries

Daily Symptom Tracking Form

Create a simple daily form that doesn't become overwhelming to complete. Include date, weather conditions (temperature, humidity, barometric pressure), sleep quality rating, and overall energy level.

Track your main symptoms using consistent scales. For example, rate heart rate symptoms, joint pain, brain fog, and digestive issues on 1-10 scales. Include space for notes about activities, triggers, or unusual events.

Record medication timing and any changes to your routine. Note meal times and any foods that might have triggered reactions. Include information about exercise, stress levels, and social activities.

Weekly and Monthly Summary Templates

Design weekly summary sheets that help identify patterns across longer periods. Calculate average symptom levels, note any correlation with weather patterns, menstrual cycles, or stress events.

Monthly summaries should track overall trends, medication effectiveness, and any major changes in your condition. Note appointments with medical providers and any treatment adjustments made during the month.

Include space for goal setting and progress tracking. Record accomplishments, challenges, and areas where you want to focus improvement efforts in the coming month.

Trigger Identification Worksheets

Create specific forms for tracking potential triggers when you suspect certain foods, activities, or environmental factors affect your symptoms. Include detailed timing information and symptom responses.

Design elimination diet tracking sheets if you're working to identify food triggers. Track what you eat, when you eat it, and any symptoms that occur within 24 hours.

Include environmental trigger tracking for factors like weather changes, air quality, chemical exposures, or seasonal allergens that might affect your symptoms.

Provider Communication Templates

New Patient Introduction Email

Develop a template for introducing yourself to new medical providers that efficiently communicates your complex medical history. Start with a brief summary of your three main conditions and how they interact.

Include your current symptom management strategies and what treatments have been most effective. Mention any treatments that have been ineffective or caused adverse reactions.

Provide a concise timeline of your diagnosis journey and current treatment team. Include contact information for your other medical providers to facilitate communication and coordination.

Appointment Preparation Email

Create a template for sending information to providers before appointments to maximize the effectiveness of your limited time together. Include your current symptom patterns, any changes since your last visit, and specific questions or concerns.

Attach your current medication list and any symptom tracking data that might be relevant to the appointment. Include information about any recent emergency department visits or urgent care needs.

List your priorities for the appointment and any specific requests, such as prescription refills, referrals, or discussion of new treatment options.

Insurance Appeal Letter Template

Develop a template for appealing insurance denials that can be customized for different situations. Include sections for documenting medical necessity, previous treatment attempts, and expected outcomes.

Provide space for attaching supporting documentation such as physician letters, medical records, and research citations that support your request.

Include templates for both initial appeals and follow-up appeals if your first request is denied.

Workplace Accommodation Request Templates

Create formal letter templates for requesting workplace accommodations under the Americans with Disabilities Act. Include clear explanations of your functional limitations and specific accommodation requests.

Provide templates for follow-up communications about accommodation effectiveness and any needed modifications. Include language that demonstrates your commitment to job performance while requesting necessary support.

Resource Directory

Professional Organizations

Medical Societies and Specialist Directories

The American Academy of Neurology maintains directories of neurologists who specialize in autonomic disorders and can provide expert POTS management. Their website includes search functions for finding specialists by geographic location and specific expertise areas.

The American College of Allergy, Asthma & Immunology provides directories of allergists and immunologists, though finding providers specifically experienced with MCAS may require additional research and phone calls to verify expertise.

The American College of Medical Genetics and Genomics offers directories of medical geneticists who can provide EDS evaluation and genetic counseling. Many geneticists have experience with connective tissue disorders and can coordinate care with other specialists.

Specialized Clinic Networks

Mayo Clinic, Cleveland Clinic, and Johns Hopkins have specialized programs for autonomic disorders that include comprehensive evaluation and treatment for POTS patients. These centers often have multidisciplinary teams familiar with trifecta conditions.

Academic medical centers frequently have genetics clinics with EDS expertise and research programs studying connective tissue disorders. University hospitals may offer access to clinical trials and cutting-edge treatments.

International Specialist Resources

The European Society of Cardiology maintains information about autonomic disorder specialists throughout Europe. International patients may find specialists with trifecta expertise in countries with advanced healthcare systems.

Canadian healthcare resources include specialized clinics in major cities like Toronto, Montreal, and Vancouver that treat complex chronic illness patients.

Patient Organizations

National Support and Advocacy Groups

Dysautonomia International provides the most comprehensive resources for POTS patients, including physician directories, research updates, educational materials, and support group information. Their website offers extensive patient education resources and advocacy tools.

The Mastocytosis Society focuses specifically on mast cell disorders and provides resources for both systemic mastocytosis and MCAS patients. They maintain research databases and support networks for patients and families.

The Ehlers-Danlos Society offers resources for all types of EDS, including educational materials, support group directories, and advocacy initiatives. They provide excellent resources for newly diagnosed patients and families.

Specialized Support Organizations

POTS UK provides resources specifically for patients in the United Kingdom, including NHS navigation assistance and UK-specific treatment information.

PoTS Australia offers support for Australian patients, including information about accessing care through the Australian healthcare system.

The European Heritable Connective Tissue Disorders Network provides resources for EDS patients throughout Europe, including specialist directories and research information.

Condition-Specific Research Organizations

The Autonomic Disorders Consortium conducts research specifically focused on POTS and other autonomic conditions. They often seek patient participants for research studies and clinical trials.

The Mastocytosis Research Fund supports research into mast cell disorders and provides funding for studies that may benefit MCAS patients.

Research Resources

Medical Literature Access

PubMed provides free access to abstracts of medical research papers and many full-text articles about POTS, MCAS, and EDS. Learning to use effective search terms helps you find relevant research about your conditions.

Google Scholar offers another way to access medical research and often provides links to free full-text versions of research papers that may not be available through other sources.

Many patient advocacy organizations maintain research databases with summaries of important studies written in patient-friendly language.

Understanding Medical Research

Learn to identify different types of studies and their relative strength of evidence. Systematic reviews and meta-analyses provide the strongest evidence, followed by randomized controlled trials, observational studies, and case reports.

Understand basic statistical concepts that appear in medical research, such as confidence intervals, p-values, and effect sizes. Many patient organizations provide guides for interpreting medical research.

Be cautious about applying research results to your specific situation, especially when studies involve small numbers of participants or don't specifically address your combination of conditions.

Clinical Trial Information

ClinicalTrials.gov maintains databases of current and planned research studies, including trials specifically for POTS, MCAS, and EDS patients. You can search by condition, location, and trial status.

Understand the different phases of clinical trials and what participation might involve. Early phase trials test safety while later phase trials compare new treatments to existing standards of care.

Consider both risks and benefits of clinical trial participation, including the time commitment required and potential for receiving placebo treatments.

Financial Resources

Patient Assistance Programs

Most major pharmaceutical companies offer patient assistance programs that provide free or reduced-cost medications for patients who meet income requirements. These programs often cover expensive specialty medications used for chronic illness treatment.

GoodRx and similar services provide discount programs for both prescription and over-the-counter medications. These can be particularly helpful for medications not covered by insurance.

RxAssist.org maintains a comprehensive database of patient assistance programs and provides guidance for applying to multiple programs efficiently.

Grant and Financial Aid Programs

The HealthWell Foundation provides grants to help with insurance premiums, copayments, and other medical expenses for patients with chronic illnesses.

Patient Advocate Foundation offers both direct financial assistance and help navigating insurance and medical billing issues.

Local community foundations may offer medical expense grants for residents facing financial hardship due to chronic illness.

Insurance Navigation Resources

Healthcare.gov provides information about health insurance options and subsidies that may be available to help with premium costs.

State insurance commissioner offices often provide assistance with insurance disputes and can help resolve coverage denials or billing problems.

Legal aid organizations may provide free or low-cost assistance with disability applications and insurance appeals.

Technology Tools

Recommended Apps

Symptom Tracking Applications

MyRA offers comprehensive symptom tracking specifically designed for people with chronic illnesses. The app allows customization of tracked symptoms and provides graphing and reporting features that help identify patterns.

Symple Symptom Tracker provides simple, user-friendly symptom logging with the ability to track multiple symptoms, medications, and triggers simultaneously. The app generates reports that can be shared with healthcare providers.

ArthritisPower, developed by CatchMyPain, includes features specifically designed for chronic pain tracking and includes weather correlation features that may be helpful for EDS patients.

Medication Management Apps

Medisafe provides medication reminders, drug interaction checking, and pill tracking features. The app can send alerts to family members if medications are missed and includes features for tracking side effects.

Pillpack (now part of Amazon Pharmacy) offers both an app and physical packaging services that organize medications by dose time, reducing the complexity of managing multiple medications.

MyTherapy combines medication reminders with symptom and mood tracking, allowing you to see correlations between medication timing and symptom patterns.

Communication and Healthcare Apps

MyChart and similar patient portal apps allow secure communication with healthcare providers, access to test results, and appointment scheduling from most major healthcare systems.

HIPAA-compliant messaging apps like TigerConnect allow secure communication with healthcare providers who use these platforms.

Telehealth apps from providers like Teladoc or Doxy.me enable virtual medical appointments, which can be particularly valuable for people with mobility limitations or transportation challenges.

Wearable Device Guide

Heart Rate Monitoring Devices

Chest strap heart rate monitors like those from Polar or Garmin provide the most accurate heart rate data during activity and can help POTS patients monitor their responses to exercise and daily activities.

Smartwatches like Apple Watch or Fitbit provide continuous heart rate monitoring and can alert you to unusual heart rate patterns. Some models include irregular heart rhythm detection that may be helpful for POTS monitoring.

Consider devices that allow you to set custom heart rate alerts based on your specific POTS management needs rather than using standard fitness-based alert levels.

Sleep and Activity Tracking

Fitness trackers with sleep monitoring capabilities can help identify sleep pattern disruptions that may correlate with symptom severity. Look for devices that track sleep stages and provide sleep quality scores.

Activity trackers help monitor daily step counts, energy expenditure, and movement patterns that can inform pacing strategies and activity modification.

Some devices include stress monitoring features that use heart rate variability to assess autonomic nervous system function, which may be particularly relevant for POTS patients.

Blood Pressure and Other Monitoring

Home blood pressure monitors with smartphone connectivity allow easy tracking of blood pressure patterns that can be shared with healthcare providers monitoring POTS treatment.

Pulse oximeters can be helpful for monitoring oxygen saturation, particularly if you experience breathing symptoms or exercise intolerance.

Smart scales that track weight trends can help monitor fluid retention patterns that may be relevant to POTS management.

Online Resources

Educational Websites and Databases

The Cleveland Clinic and Mayo Clinic websites provide reliable, comprehensive information about POTS, MCAS, and EDS written for both patients and healthcare providers.

WebMD and Healthline offer basic information about chronic illness management, though their content about rare conditions like MCAS may be limited.

The National Institutes of Health (NIH) website includes research updates and detailed information about rare diseases, including comprehensive information about EDS types.

Online Learning Platforms

Coursera and edX offer courses about healthcare, medical research, and chronic illness management that can help you become a more informed patient and advocate.

Khan Academy provides free courses about basic biology, anatomy, and health topics that can help you better understand your conditions and treatments.

Patient advocacy organizations often provide webinar series and online educational events specifically designed for people with chronic illnesses.

Digital Health Platforms

PatientsLikeMe allows you to connect with other patients, track symptoms, and contribute to research studies about your conditions.

Smart Patients provides moderated online communities focused on specific medical conditions with emphasis on sharing reliable health information.

Mighty Networks hosts various chronic illness communities with features for private messaging, group discussions, and resource sharing.

These appendices and resources provide practical tools and information sources that support effective chronic illness management. Regular review and updating of these resources ensures that you have current, relevant information available when you need it most. The combination of prepared templates, reliable information sources, and appropriate technology tools creates a foundation for successful long-term management of complex chronic conditions.

References

1. Dysautonomia International. POTS and Sleep Disorders: Understanding the Connection. 2023.

2. Freeman R, et al. Orthostatic hypotension: JACC Scientific Statement. Journal of the American College of Cardiology. 2011;58(15):1549-1560.

3. Moldofsky H. Sleep and pain. Sleep Medicine Reviews. 2001;5(5):385-396.

4. Theoharides TC, et al. Mast cells and inflammation. Biochimica et Biophysica Acta. 2012;1822(1):21-33.

5. Tinkle B, et al. Hypermobile Ehlers-Danlos syndrome (a.k.a. Ehlers-Danlos syndrome Type III and Ehlers-Danlos syndrome hypermobility type): Clinical description and natural history. American Journal of Medical Genetics Part C. 2017;175(1):48-69.

6. Boris JR, et al. Youth with chronic fatigue syndrome and orthostatic intolerance: Clinical presentation and response to treatment. Journal of Pediatrics. 2019;212:111-117.

7. Akin C, et al. Diagnosis and classification of mastocytosis: Consensus proposals from the European Competence Network on Mastocytosis. Leukemia Research. 2001;25(7):603-625.

8. Castori M, et al. A framework for the classification of joint hypermobility and related conditions. American Journal of Medical Genetics Part C. 2017;175(1):148-157.

9. Stewart JM. Common syndromes of orthostatic intolerance. Pediatrics. 2013;131(5):968-980.

10. Valent P, et al. Definitions, criteria and global classification of mast cell disorders with special reference to mast cell activation syndromes. Journal of Allergy and Clinical Immunology. 2012;129(6):1404-1414.

11. Malfait F, et al. The 2017 international classification of the Ehlers-Danlos syndromes. American Journal of Medical Genetics Part C. 2017;175(1):8-26.

12. Sheldon RS, et al. 2015 Heart Rhythm Society expert consensus statement on the diagnosis and treatment of postural tachycardia syndrome. Heart Rhythm. 2015;12(6):e41-e63.

13. Fedorowski A, et al. Orthostatic hypotension: management of a complex, but common, medical problem. Circulation: Arrhythmia and Electrophysiology. 2019;12(3):e007750.

14. Freeman R, et al. Consensus statement on the definition of orthostatic hypotension, neurally mediated syncope and the postural tachycardia syndrome. Clinical Autonomic Research. 2011;21(2):69-72.

15. Church MK, Church DS. Pharmacology of antihistamines. Australian Prescriber. 2013;36(2):50-56.

16. Zampeli E, et al. Treatment of mast cell activation disease: A systematic review. Journal of Allergy and Clinical Immunology. 2014;134(4):979-980.

17. Castells M, et al. Diagnosis and treatment of anaphylaxis: An updated practice parameter. Journal of Allergy and Clinical Immunology. 2020;145(4):1082-1123.

18. Reiter R, et al. Guidelines for the diagnosis and management of mast cell activation syndrome (MCAS). Journal of Allergy and Clinical Immunology: In Practice. 2020;8(4):1368-1386.

19. Derry S, et al. Pregabalin for neuropathic pain in adults. Cochrane Database of Systematic Reviews. 2019;1:CD007076.

20. Wehling M. Non-steroidal anti-inflammatory drug use in chronic pain conditions with special emphasis on the elderly and patients with relevant comorbidities: Management and mitigation of risks and adverse effects. European Journal of Clinical Pharmacology. 2014;70(10):1159-1172.

21. See S, Ginzburg R. Choosing a skeletal muscle relaxant. American Family Physician. 2008;78(3):365-370.

22. Boullata JI, et al. Drug-nutrient interactions: A broad view with implications for practice. Journal of the Academy of Nutrition and Dietetics. 2012;112(4):506-517.

23. Lynch T, Price A. The effect of cytochrome P450 metabolism on drug response, interactions, and adverse effects. American Family Physician. 2007;76(3):391-396.

24. Yu LX, Kopelman BI. The evolution of FDA's generic drug bioequivalence program: A regulatory perspective. AAPS Journal. 2017;19(6):1561-1567.

25. Guyatt GH, et al. GRADE: An emerging consensus on rating quality of evidence and strength of recommendations. BMJ. 2008;336(7650):924-926.

26. Calder PC. Omega-3 fatty acids and inflammatory processes: From molecules to man. Biochemical Society Transactions. 2017;45(5):1105-1115.

27. de Baaij JH, et al. Magnesium in man: Implications for health and disease. Physiological Reviews. 2015;95(1):1-46.

28. Holick MF. Vitamin D deficiency. New England Journal of Medicine. 2007;357(3):266-281.

29. Zhai J, et al. Coenzyme Q10 in the treatment of mitochondrial myopathies. A multi-center double-blind trial. European Journal of Neurology. 2017;24(2):370-379.

30. Mlcek J, et al. Quercetin and its anti-allergic immune response. Molecules. 2016;21(5):623.

31. Johnston CS, et al. Vitamin C supplementation slightly improves physical activity levels and reduces cold incidence in men with marginal vitamin C status: A randomized controlled trial. Nutrients. 2014;6(7):2572-2583.

32. Maintz L, Novak N. Histamine and histamine intolerance. American Journal of Clinical Nutrition. 2007;85(5):1185-1196.

33. Sigurjonsdottir HA, et al. Is blood pressure commonly raised by moderate consumption of liquorice? Journal of Human Hypertension. 2001;15(8):549-552.

34. Brownlie T 4th, et al. Tissue iron deficiency without anemia impairs adaptation in endurance capacity after aerobic training in previously untrained women. American Journal of Clinical Nutrition. 2004;79(3):437-443.

35. Goyal M, et al. Meditation programs for psychological stress and well-being: A systematic review and meta-analysis. JAMA Internal Medicine. 2014;174(3):357-368.

36. Jacobson E. Progressive relaxation: A physiological and clinical investigation of muscular states and their significance in psychology and medical practice. Chicago: University of Chicago Press; 1938.

37. Ma X, et al. The effect of diaphragmatic breathing on attention, negative affect and stress in healthy adults. Frontiers in Psychology. 2017;8:874.

38. Lehrer PM, Gevirtz R. Heart rate variability biofeedback: How and why does it work? Frontiers in Psychology. 2014;5:756.

39. Thayer JF, Lane RD. Claude Bernard and the heart-brain connection: Further elaboration of a model of neurovisceral integration. Neuroscience & Biobehavioral Reviews. 2009;33(2):81-88.

40. Cramer H, et al. A systematic review and meta-analysis of yoga for low back pain. Clinical Journal of Pain. 2013;29(5):450-460.

41. Wayne PM, et al. Effect of tai chi on cognitive performance in older adults: Systematic review and meta-analysis. Journal of the American Geriatrics Society. 2014;62(1):25-39.

42. Field T. Massage therapy research review. Complementary Therapies in Clinical Practice. 2016;24:19-31.

43. Ernst E, White AR. Acupuncture for back pain: A meta-analysis of randomized controlled trials. Archives of Internal Medicine. 2001;161(11):1081-1088.

44. Green C, et al. A systematic review of craniosacral therapy: Biological plausibility, assessment reliability and clinical effectiveness. BMJ Open. 2019;9(8):e029721.

45. Johnson MI, et al. Transcutaneous electrical nerve stimulation (TENS) for fibromyalgia in adults. Cochrane Database of Systematic Reviews. 2017;10:CD012172.

46. Compression stockings for preventing recurrence of venous ulcers. Cochrane Database of Systematic Reviews. 2018;7:CD002303.

47. Henderson L, et al. St John's wort (Hypericum perforatum): Drug interactions and clinical outcomes. British Journal of Clinical Pharmacology. 2002;54(4):349-356.

48. Campbell RL, et al. Emergency department diagnosis and treatment of anaphylaxis: A practice parameter.

Annals of Allergy, Asthma & Immunology. 2014;113(6):599-608.

49. Simons FE, et al. World allergy organization guidelines for the assessment and management of anaphylaxis. World Allergy Organization Journal. 2011;4(2):13-37.

50. Americans with Disabilities Act of 1990, 42 U.S.C. § 12101 et seq. (1990).

51. Goering S. Rethinking disability: The social model of disability and chronic disease. Current Reviews in Musculoskeletal Medicine. 2015;8(2):134-138.

52. Job Accommodation Network. Accommodation and Compliance Series: Employees with Chronic Fatigue Syndrome. Morgantown, WV: Job Accommodation Network; 2021.

53. Beatty PW, et al. Access to health care services among people with chronic or disabling conditions: Patterns and predictors. Archives of Physical Medicine and Rehabilitation. 2003;84(10):1417-1425.

54. Charmaz K. Good Days, Bad Days: The Self in Chronic Illness and Time. New Brunswick, NJ: Rutgers University Press; 1991.

55. Stanton AL, et al. The adaptive potential of coping with cancer diagnosis and treatment: A review of existing evidence. Social Science & Medicine. 2007;65(11):2217-2228.

56. Folkman S. Stress, coping, and hope. Psycho-Oncology. 2010;19(9):901-908.

57. Tedeschi RG, Calhoun LG. Posttraumatic growth: Conceptual foundations and empirical evidence. Psychological Inquiry. 2004;15(1):1-18.

58. Hayes SC, et al. Acceptance and Commitment Therapy: The Process and Practice of Mindful Change. New York: Guilford Press; 2011.

59. Beck AT, et al. Cognitive Therapy of Depression. New York: Guilford Press; 1979.

www.ingramcontent.com/pod-product-compliance
Lightning Source LLC
Chambersburg PA
CBHW050502270326
41927CB00009B/1863